Pilun Piyasirivej

Web Usability Evaluation

Pilun Piyasirivej

Web Usability Evaluation

Using a Contingent Heuristic Approach and Eye
Gaze Tracking for the Usability Evaluation of
Web Sites

VDM Verlag Dr. Müller

Imprint

Bibliographic information by the German National Library: The German National Library lists this publication at the German National Bibliography; detailed bibliographic information is available on the Internet at http://dnb.d-nb.de.

Cover image: www.purestockx.com

Publisher:
VDM Verlag Dr. Müller Aktiengesellschaft & Co. KG , Dudweiler Landstr. 125 a, 66123 Saarbrücken, Germany,
Phone +49 681 9100-698, Fax +49 681 9100-988,
Email: info@vdm-verlag.de

Zugl.: Murdoch, Murdoch University, Diss., 2004

Produced in USA and UK by:
Lightning Source Inc., La Vergne, Tennessee, USA
Lightning Source UK Ltd., Milton Keynes, UK
BookSurge LLC, 5341 Dorchester Road, Suite 16, North Charleston, SC 29418, USA

ISBN: 978-3-639-01516-4

*This book is dedicated to the memory of
Professor Magid Igbaria (1958-2002),
my professor and mentor, who contributed
so much to information systems research.
You will always be remembered.*

Contents

1

Overview

1.1 Introduction

This book is the culmination of the 18-month research study undertaken at the School of Information Technology, Murdoch University, Western Australia. It describes a research study in Human-Computer Interaction (HCI), within the information technology discipline. Although it is often regarded that information technology as a field is still young, it is closely related to one of the most well-established disciplines: *information science*. The relationship between information technology and information science is described as follows:

> Information science is a field devoted to scientific inquiry and professional practice addressing the problems of effective communication of knowledge and knowledge records among humans in the context of social, institutional and/or individual uses of and needs for information. In addressing these problems of particular interest is taking as much advantage as possible of the modern information technology. [...] Information science is inexorably connected to information technology. A technological imperative is compelling and constraining the evolution of information science, as is the evolution of information society. (Saracevic, 1995)

One can argue that definitions of information science are inconsistent (depending on the source) and change over time. This is mainly because information science is a living discipline that is still evolving. Thus, there is no clear-cut boundary between what is considered information science and what is not. Nevertheless, the above definition of information science is appropriate and valid for the past decade (and probably for the next decade as well) because during the 1990s and 2000s, information technology is involved more often than not in the information science research area.

Information technology as a field is very comprehensive; it includes several sub-areas, e.g. software development, artificial intelligence, bioinformatics, etc. This book concentrates on the area of Human-Computer Interaction and usability evaluation. The justification for this selection will be presented in the following chapter.

All of the research work in this study was carried out using facilities within the Murdoch University campus, and all of the participants involved in the experiments conducted as part of the study were Murdoch university undergraduate students. This research study consists mainly of a literature review and behavioural experiments. Both quantitative and qualitative research approaches were utilised to produce synergistic power and gain thorough understanding regarding the topic addressed: *Using a contingent heuristic approach and eye gaze tracking for the usability evaluation of Web sites.*

It has been widely accepted that the World Wide Web (shortened "Web" or WWW) is by far the most popular medium used by today's professionals and novices alike, for various reasons that will be discussed in Chapter 2. Many aspects of the Web have been investigated by scholars in various fields, one of which is the usability of Web sites. There are various issues regarding the usability of Web sites, and many of them have already been investigated within the last decade. Nevertheless, there have been very few studies that address the following usability evaluation techniques: *(1) contingent heuristic approach;* and *(2) eye gaze tracking.* This research study utilised these two techniques and evaluated their effectiveness and efficiency, with regard to the usability evaluation of Web sites. By investigating these two emerging techniques in further detail, this book makes them more widely known to scholars and professional Web site developers, as alternative means for Web site usability evaluation.

There are several criteria by which Web sites could be selected for usability evaluation. After investigating various possibilities, this study concentrates on the distinction between Flash-based and HTML-based Web sites. The main reason for this selection is that during the past few years, there has been increasing controversy regarding whether Flash or HTML Web sites provide higher usability to users. However, very few studies were done previously regarding this issue. Hence this book is among the first of its kind to present the comparative study of Flash and HTML Web sites focusing on usability.

1.2   Structure of Book

The structure of this book is organised in a storytelling, chronological manner. It takes you through the research journey that starts with an overview of Human-Computer Interaction as a field, usability evaluation methods and techniques, and their application to the Web (Chapter 2). Then, the heuristic approaches, consisting of heuristic evaluation and questionnaire, were chosen and explored in more detail in Chapter 3, because of their relevance to the contingent heuristic approach, which itself is discussed in Chapter 4. This chapter also introduces you to the Website Usability Contingent Evaluation Tool (WUCET), which is one possible implementation of the contingent heuristic approach.

The journey continues with the discussion of eye gaze tracking as a method for Web site usability evaluation (Chapter 5). This includes the exploration of several eye tracking systems available on the market, a literature review of previous related studies, and procedures commonly undertaken for usability evaluation using the eye gaze tracking technique. After that, the importance of Flash technology in Web site development is discussed in Chapter 6, and several research questions/hypotheses regarding the comparative usability of Flash and HTML Web sites are also proposed, in regard to several influential factors including user's gender, experience, and site purpose.

The research methods chosen in order to test these hypotheses are presented in detail in Chapter 7. It describes two phases of experiment, one of which utilises the contingent heuristic approach through WUCET questionnaires, and the other utilises the eye tracking technique with the faceLAB eye tracking system.

Results from the analyses of the questionnaires and the eye tracking experiment are presented in Chapter 8 and Chapter 9, respectively. In these two chapters, the evaluations of both WUCET and eye gaze tracking technique are also made according to users' comments regarding their experience with the experiments.

At the end of the journey (Chapter 10), several conclusions are drawn from the research outcomes in respect to the research questions, and recommendations for further research are also presented.

2

Human-Computer Interaction and Web Usability Evaluation

2.1 Introduction

Human-Computer Interaction (HCI), as its name suggests, is the study of how humans and computers interact. How to make this interaction as effective and efficient as possible is the main concern of HCI professionals, as pointed out by Long (1989, p. 5):

> Human-computer interaction comprises phenomena and a discipline which takes those phenomena as its scope. The phenomena involve systems consisting of: people—both as individuals and as social organisations; computers—both stand-alone and as networks; and their interaction. Since the systems are physical and informational, so too are their interactions. The discipline is concerned to support the optimisation of the interactions between humans and computers to perform work effectively. The concern, then, is not with the interactions in isolation. Humans use computers to do work and also have performance requirements for the work which is carried out. Interactions and their optimisation, then, need to be developed in the context of work and performance.

In essence, works in the field of HCI usually fall into one of the following domains:

1. The development of human capabilities to use machines
2. The designing and building of interfaces
3. The optimization of the performance of tasks by humans and machines
4. Usability of the interface itself
5. A better communication between human and machines (Sarmento, 2004)

If we look closer at the input and output attributes of a computer, we see that they are very powerful: anything that can be digitised in the form of bits (binary digits of 0s and 1s) can be an input or an output of a computer. Examples include, but are not limited to, text, image, sound, and electrical signal. Of course, there are some kinds of information that today cannot be digitised, such as smell and taste, but who knows about the future? Computers are getting better every day; perhaps someday we will be able to browse for perfumes on the Web and print their scents out of a machine similar to today's printer. If this dream ever comes true, then we can shop for many more things without leaving the comfort of our own homes.

Now let us look at the other side of the connection: human. Input and output mechanisms of humans are not the same as those of a computer. People take inputs mainly in the forms of sight, sound, touch, smell, and taste (collectively called the "5 senses"), while their outputs are limited to sound (voice) and body movement (e.g. handwriting, gesture, etc.) only. That is why we cannot just connect a person to a computer with a cable to transfer information. The nature of a human's input and output capabilities has forced us to adapt computers to meet the needs and limitations of humans, and this is what HCI is all about: doing the best we can to make communication between people and computers more effective, more efficient, and more successful. Flanagan, Huang, Jones, and Kasif (1997) emphasise that this can be achieved by implementing user interfaces that interact with human senses as follows:

> The sensory modalities of sight, sound, and touch are major channels for the human (senses of smell and taste being less utilized in most information management tasks). Integration of these modalities can support human judgment, but the technologies for sight (visual presentation, spatial organization, gesture, gaze tracking, image recognition), sound (speech recognition, text-to-speech synthesis, speech store-and-forward, non-speech audio), and touch (manual gesture, two-handed input, grasp, force feedback) are incompletely developed. Development of multimodal interfaces is therefore a central concern of human-centered systems.

In the early days of the computer era, the days of mainframes and punch cards, HCI may not have played an important role because most systems were computer-centred, i.e. users had to conform to the limited capabilities of computer hardware and software. In Europe, HCI came into view when the *International Journal of Man-Machine Studies* (later renamed the *International Journal of Human-Computer Studies*) was first published in 1969 in the United Kingdom. Nevertheless, it was not until March 1982 that HCI made its official debut in the United States, when the *Human Factors in Computer Systems* conference was organised by the (U.S.) National Bureau of Standards (now the National Institute of Standards and Technology) (Carroll, 2002). Since then, technology has changed, and the focus has shifted from computer-centred to human-centred systems. There are two main reasons for this: (1) the increasing number of computer users, and (2) the increasing power of computers.

The increasing number of users means that computers are not used exclusively by computer professionals (e.g. computer engineers, scientists, programmers) anymore; now they are being used by professionals in other fields (e.g. doctors, nurses, teachers, biologists) as well as the general public, including children. Thus special attention is required when a computer system, whether hardware or software, is designed and developed, since the system will be nothing more than a piece of code or plastic if people cannot use it. From a scientific and social viewpoint, systems that nobody wants to use fail because they do not contribute any value to mankind. From a business viewpoint, they fail because they will not sell. That is why the term "usability" has emerged and is now the focus of the worldwide computer industry. More often than not, usability is used synonymously with HCI. Carroll (2002, p. xxvii) concisely defines HCI as *"the study and the practice of usability."* He also points out that *"it is about understanding and creating software and other technology that people will want to use, will be able to use, and will find effective when used."*

The other important factor that enables us to create user-friendly systems is the increase in the computer's power, which includes faster execution time, larger storage capacity, and the most important of all, a higher level of intelligence. Thanks to the ever-growing field of artificial intelligence, computers are now smarter than ever before, as was shown by IBM Deep Blue Supercomputer's victory over the world's greatest human chess player, Garry Kasparov, on May 11, 1997. This event increased the concern that humans may soon lose their power to machines. From HCI's perspective, though, there is no fear because as computers are more intelligent, they can greatly reduce the burden that users have to bear when using their computers. This can be seen in as simple a thing as a personal computer (PC). Twenty years ago most PCs exploited text-based operating systems and applications; users had to memorise text commands and type them in correctly to get the desired results. However, these procedures have gradually changed over the years. We can see that most PCs today use graphical user interface systems. Users of these systems do not need to memorise any text commands; all they have to do to get their work done is point and click at items on the screen. On some systems, users may also use their voice or handwriting to communicate with their PCs.

2.2   HCI Research: Past, Present, and Future

HCI is a young and interdisciplinary field; it exploits knowledge and skills from many well-established disciplines including computer science, cognitive psychology, social and organisational psychology, ergonomics and human factors, linguistics, artificial intelligence, philosophy, sociology and anthropology, and engineering and design (Preece, Rogers, Sharp, Benyon, Holland, and Carey, 1994, p. 48). No one research project can explore all of these disciplines in depth, but as many of them gather together, they can build the field of HCI to be as solid as any other field. Although HCI has been regarded as a field since the early 1980s, its roots can be traced back to four independent threads of technical development from the 1960s and 1970s:

1. Prototyping and iterative development from software engineering
2. Software psychology and human factors of computing systems
3. User interface software from computer graphics
4. Models, theories, and frameworks from cognitive science (Carroll, 2002, p. xxvii)

These four roots are important as they are still the foundation of the HCI field even now. Over the past two decades, there have been countless research projects contributing to the field of HCI; Table 2.1 summarises most of the HCI research areas and their progress over the years.

Table 2.1   HCI research areas

	Past	Present	Future
HCI theoretical framework (Sutcliffe, 2000)	Goals, Operators, Methods, and Selection (GOMS)	Soar ACT-R Executive-Process Interactive Control (EPIC)	Cognitive Task Model (CTM) Kaur's model Task-artifact theory
User interface	Text-based	Graphical Multimedia	Invisible (Norman, 1998)
Input method	Keyboard Mouse	Voice Handwriting	Eye gaze Facial expression Gesture
Interaction scheme	Mass production	Mass customisation Localisation	Personalisation (Turk and Badii, 2001)
System development	Computer-centred	Task-centred	Human-centred
Web platform	PCs	Handhelds Mobiles/Wireless Application Protocol (WAP)	Anywhere
Computer-based learning	Computer-Aided Instruction (CAI)	E-learning	Anywhere
Computers at work	Stand-alone	Internet/Intranet E-mail	Groupware Computer-Supported Cooperative Work (CSCW)
Other topics	Social/cultural issues Accessibility Ethics		

During these years, several organisations devoted entirely to HCI have also emerged, along with a number of specialist journals and conferences. Some prominent examples of these organisations, journals, and conferences are shown in Table 2.2.

Table 2.2   Major HCI organisations, journals, and conferences

Organisations	Journals	Conferences
Association for Computing Machinery (ACM) Special Interest Group on Computer-Human Interaction (SIGCHI)	ACM Transactions on Computer-Human Interaction (TOCHI)	Conference On Human Factors In Computing Systems (CHI)
		Annual ACM Symposium on User Interface Software and Technology (UIST)
Association for Information Systems (AIS) Special Interest Group on Human-Computer Interaction (SIGHCI)	-	Americas Conference on Information Systems (AMCIS) Track on Human-Computer Interaction Studies in MIS
		Annual Workshop on HCI Research in MIS
British HCI Group	Interacting with Computers: The Interdisciplinary Journal of Human-Computer Interaction	British HCI Group Annual Conference (HCI)
Ergonomics Society	Ergonomics: The Official Journal of the Ergonomics Society and the International Ergonomics Association	Ergonomics Society Annual Conference
European Association of Cognitive Ergonomics (EACE)	-	Annual Conference of the European Association of Cognitive Ergonomics (EACE)
Human Factors and Ergonomics Society (HFES)	Human Factors: The Journal of the Human Factors and Ergonomics Society	Human Factors and Ergonomics Society Annual Meeting
International Federation for Information Processing (IFIP) Technical Committee on Human-Computer Interaction	-	IFIP International Conference on Human-Computer Interaction (INTERACT)
		IFIP Working Conference on Engineering for Human-Computer Interaction (EHCI)
Usability Professionals' Association (UPA)	International Journal of Usability Studies	Usability Professionals' Association Annual Conference
-	-	International Conference on Human-Computer Interaction (HCI International)

Publishers	Journals	
Elsevier	International Journal of Human-Computer Studies	
Lawrence Erlbaum Associates	Human-Computer Interaction: A Journal of Theoretical, Empirical, and Methodological Issues of User Science and of System Design	
	International Journal of Human-Computer Interaction	
Taylor & Francis	Behaviour & Information Technology	

Karat and Karat (2003) categorise papers in the field of HCI into four categories: *system* (papers about systems intended to enhance some human activity), *method* (papers about methods for the development of systems), *usage analysis* (papers offering analysis of some activity employing technology), and *user interface comparison* (papers comparing two or more design approaches for systems to accomplish some task). In addition, Karat and Karat (2003) also compare the number of papers in each category presented in early conferences (CHI'83, INTERACT'84, CHI'85) and recent ones (CHI'01, INTERACT 2001, CHI'02), as shown in Table 2.3.

Table 2.3   Analysis of paper topic distribution in early and recent ACM SIGCHI and IFIP INTERACT conferences (Karat and Karat, 2003)

Paper Topics	Percentage of Papers in CHI'83, INTERACT'84, and CHI'85 (n=207)	Percentage of Papers in CHI'01, INTERACT 2001, and CHI'02 (n=214)
System	17	35
Method	15	6
Usage Analysis	26	27
UI Comparison	14	20
Others	28	12

Although the distribution of papers in each category may have changed over the last two decades, e.g. an increase in the number of papers discussing new or unique systems and a decrease in the number of papers about methods, right now HCI is still one of the most active and fruitful fields in the computer industry because it has a great impact on everyone's life, as we can see from the number of HCI research projects that is growing every day. The next section discusses usability evaluation, which is one of the most important areas within the field of HCI.

2.3 Definitions of Usability

In the previous section, we have seen that usability is indeed one of the core issues of human-computer interaction. It can be defined concisely as the ease-of-use of a particular hardware or software system. More detailed definitions of the term "usability" can be found in many HCI textbooks, including Shackel and Richardson (1991, p. 24):

> Usability of a system or equipment is the capability in human functional terms to be used easily and effectively by the specified range of users, given specified training and user support, to fulfil the specified range of tasks, within the specified range of environmental scenarios.

The importance of usability in today's computing environment is expressed clearly by Maxwell (2002, p. 193) as follows:

> During the past 20 years, computers have been vigorously transferred from laboratories and central data processing centers, in which only skilled experts used them, to offices and homes, for use by people who need to perform a wide range of tasks that can be assisted by personal computing technologies. However, this expanded group of computer users was not necessarily trained in computer technology. The usability needs of these new computer

users propelled the growth of HCI as a discipline of study and focused its primary goal on making computers easier to use.

Usability cannot be measured on an absolute scale because it not only depends on a particular system, but also depends on a particular user of that system as well. For example, UNIX, a text-based operating system, may not be considered usable by novice computer users or users who prefer a graphical user interface, but it is very well usable by computer professionals or experienced users. In addition to personal preference and experience, the issue of whether users are more of "verbalisers" or "imagers" (i.e. having different cognitive styles: a tendency to process information in either words or images) might as well influence the perceived usability of a software system (Riding, 1991). Another example is a video game system, which is targeted towards a younger audience, and is considered one of the most successful inventions of all time, despite the fact that most adults do not buy it (except for their children) or even try it. Nowadays more personalisation is demanded by users, so it is almost impossible to design or develop a system for a universal audience (i.e. a system that works for everybody). Hence, when the usability of any particular system is discussed, it is implied that the usability in discussion means the usability of that system towards a target audience, unless there is no specific target for that system (which is very unlikely).

Although users play an important role in usability measurement, they are not the only factor involved. There are also many other factors that can affect the usability of a particular system. These factors are collectively called "context of use," which includes:

- Environmental factors: physical conditions such as space, time, temperature, noise
- Organizational factors: social network [within the organisation], management and organizational pressures, and work processes
- Technical/system factors: network connectivity, system configuration, system stability
- Broad social factors: cosmesis[1], family conflicts, career aspirations, economy, ethical standards (Usability First, 2002)

2.4   Usability Evaluation Methods and Techniques

The evaluation of usability can be done in a number of different ways. We can evaluate the usability of software components (user interfaces), the usability of hardware components (ergonomics), or the combination of both. As far as information technology as a field is concerned, information technologists usually conduct research in the area of user interface usability and leave the study of hardware usability to computer/electrical engineers and industrial designers. For that reason, from now on only the usability of user interfaces will be discussed in this book.

---

[1] The effect that the appearance of a device has on the perception of the person who is using it; it's "fashion statement". The degree to which the user can feel attractive and socially acceptable in using the device.

We may feel that the usability of many kinds of software (e.g. operating system, word processing, etc.) has improved dramatically over the past decade, but how can we prove that? Sometimes we might want to compare the usability of two or more user interfaces. How can we do that? Obviously, we need some evaluation methods and techniques in order to measure the usability of various user interfaces available on the market or under development. Usually, software usability evaluation can be undertaken either by the company that develops software itself or by any other company that specialises in usability testing. Two different forms of usability evaluation exist: *formative evaluation* and *summative evaluation* (Theng and Marsden, 1998). Formative evaluation is an evaluation of an unfinished user interface, and aims to expose usability problems that exist in the current iteration, while summative evaluation takes place after the implementation of an interface or system, and is designed to determine whether the design goals were achieved (Watson, 2001, p. 30). Figure 2.1 visually describes the nature of formative and summative evaluation.

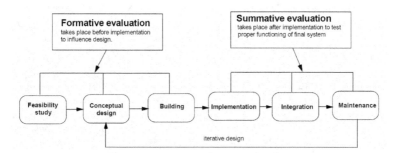

Figure 2.1   Formative and summative evaluation (Theng and Marsden, 1998)

Formative and summative evaluation stages are usually joined by iterative design because the main objective of usability evaluation is that the user interface in consideration can be improved iteratively according to the evaluation results until the client or the user of the system is satisfied.

Prototyping is a key to the evaluation of user interfaces (especially during formative stages) because evaluation of a prototype provides quick feedback from the users, so that the design of user interfaces can be easily changed and their usability can be rapidly improved even before the actual implementation takes place. Furthermore, changes during the prototyping phase do not incur as much cost as changes that occur after implementation. There are four forms of prototype, as classified by Vossen and Maguire (1998):

1. Paper prototype, which can be developed quickly and changed easily
2. Video simulation showing the concept behind the system
3. Computer-based prototype or simulation of the system concept, produced in software

4. Simulation of the system, the interface being controlled by a person, acting as the system and responding to user input (known as "Wizard of Oz" simulation)

The benefits and limitations of these prototyping methods can be found in Appendix 2A. It should also be noted that although many prototyping methods exist, only two of them are most frequently used: *paper prototyping* and *computer-based (software) prototyping*. Software prototypes are advantageous in that they have more features and are more similar to the finished interfaces than paper prototypes, while paper prototypes are cheaper to produce. Software developers have a tendency to overlook paper prototyping and start developing software prototypes from the very beginning. However, experts suggest that paper prototypes should be constructed before any programming is attempted (Cooper, 1994). Laura Arlov (in Society for Technical Communication, 2004) also suggests some of the advantages of paper-based prototypes as follows:

- Since the prototypes don't look real to customers, they are not so likely to create unrealistic expectations.
- You get more useful comments when you work with a paper prototype (more about the task, less about how things look).
- A design you've invested minutes to create has a looser grip on your ego than one on which you've spent hours, allowing you to keep a more open mind to changes and suggestions.

After prototypes have been created, it is often necessary to evaluate their usability in order to find ways to maximise the ease of use of the software. There are a number of methods and techniques that can be used to evaluate user interfaces, including:

- **Expert walkthrough (heuristic evaluation),** which is the process of letting usability experts examine a user interface and provide comments or concerns based on their experience (so-called "heuristics"). A walkthrough can be either structured (i.e. covering all possible scenarios) or unstructured (i.e. letting experts try out software on their own without forcing them to cover all possible scenarios). Usability expertise can be formalised via a list of heuristics (or dimensions) of usability. The most prominent example of usability heuristics is probably the one proposed by Nielsen (1994a) as reproduced in Appendix 2B.
- **Guidelines checklist,** which is commonly used instead of an expert walkthrough in the case where no expert is available or it costs too much to hire an expert. After software or a user interface has been developed, it can be compared to usability guidelines and checked for conformity. The check can be performed by the developer or designer, and if their user interface does not conform to guidelines, they can redesign or make changes according to guidelines in order to increase the usability of their user interface. Most usability guidelines are derived from experts' experience, so in a way, a guidelines checklist is a heuristic evaluation without experts involved. Common usability guidelines can be found in many books and also on the Web. One example is the GNOME Human Interface Guidelines (HIG) (GNOME, 2003).

- **Cognitive walkthrough,** which is a way of figuring out how people think and react when they use the system for the very first time ("learning by doing"). Cognitive walkthrough is a usability evaluation method based on cognitive theory, for example, the theory called CE+ proposed by Polson and Lewis (1990). According to the CE+ theory, when people interact with the system, they typically perform the following steps:

  1. The user sets a goal to be accomplished with the system (for example, "check spelling of this document").
  2. The user searches the interface for currently available actions (menu items, buttons, command-line inputs, etc.).
  3. The user selects the action that seems likely to make progress toward the goal.
  4. The user performs the selected action and evaluates the system's feedback for evidence that progress is being made toward the current goal. (Rieman, Franzke, and Redmiles, 1995, p. 387)

  Therefore, when a cognitive walkthrough is performed, the following questions must be asked by the evaluator:

  1. Will the user try to achieve the right effect?
  2. Will the user notice that the correct action is available?
  3. Will the user associate the correct action with the effect trying to be achieved?
  4. If the correct action is performed, will the user see that progress is being made toward solution of the task? (Wharton, Rieman, Lewis, and Polson, 1994, p. 112)

- **Observing user behaviour,** which can be carried out in a number of different ways, including fixed laboratory testing, portable laboratory testing, remote usability testing, and automated usability testing (Chang and Dillon, 1997). Moreover, observation can exploit common techniques such as keystroke recording, mouse movement monitoring, and videotaping, or emerging techniques such as eye movement and facial expression monitoring. Regardless of place or technique chosen, there are common steps that have to be undertaken while observing users. Gomoll (1990, pp. 87-90) suggests ten steps as follows:

  1. Set up the observation.
  2. Describe the purpose of the observation (in general terms).
  3. Tell the user that it's OK to quit at any time.
  4. Talk about and demonstrate the equipment in the room.
  5. Explain how to "think aloud."
  6. Explain that you will not provide help.
  7. Describe the tasks and introduce the product.
  8. Ask if there are any questions before you start; then begin the observation.
  9. Conclude the observation.
  10. Use the results.

- **Questionnaire,** which is a traditional way of getting user's feedback, can be used to evaluate usability of the system. Usually, selected users are asked to fill in a questionnaire regarding their attitude towards the system. Evaluators can develop a questionnaire using their own set of questions or choose from various questionnaires available on the market. The Software Usability Measurement Inventory (SUMI) is an example of a usability questionnaire commercially available from the Human Factors Research Group (HFRG) in Ireland. It includes 50 items to be completed by a user on a three-point scale (agree, don't know, disagree) and it produces measures on five scales of usability: efficiency, affect, helpfulness, control, and learnability (Kirakowski, 1994). The values given by users for a particular user interface are compared with a database of past results to evaluate whether this user interface is better or worse than average, and by how much.

We have seen that there are several usability evaluation methods and techniques available, but which one to choose? The answer depends on many factors and thus cannot be answered precisely without an in-depth investigation. However, there are a number of research papers that attempt to compare some of the methods in general, such as the one by Jeffries, Miller, Wharton, and Uyeda (1991) which compares four different techniques: heuristic evaluation, software guidelines, cognitive walkthroughs, and usability testing (observing user behaviour). The results of that study are summarised in Table 2.4.

Table 2.4   Comparison of four usability evaluation techniques (Jeffries et al., 1991, p. 123)

Techniques	Advantages	Disadvantages
Heuristic evaluation	• Identifies many more problems • Identifies more serious problems • Low cost	• Requires UI^2 expertise • Requires several evaluators
Usability testing	• Identifies serious and recurring problems • Avoids low-priority problems	• Requires UI expertise • High cost • Misses consistency problems
Guidelines	• Identifies recurring and general problems • Can be used by software developers	• Misses some severe problems
Cognitive walkthrough	• Helps define users' goals and assumptions • Can be used by software developers	• Needs task definition methodology • Tedious • Misses general and recurring problems

Apart from the work of Jeffries et al., Holzinger (2005) provides a useful comparison of usability evaluation techniques. Holzinger divides usability evaluation methods into two groups: *inspection methods* (without end users) and *test methods* (with end

---

[2] User Interface

users). Inspection methods include heuristic evaluation, cognitive walkthrough, and action analysis (keystroke-level analysis); test methods include thinking aloud, field observation, and questionnaires. Table 2.5 shows the results of this study.

Table 2.5   Comparison of usability evaluation techniques (Holzinger, 2005)

	Inspection Methods			Test Methods		
	Heuristic Evaluation	**Cognitive Walk-through**	**Action Analysis**	**Thinking Aloud**	**Field Obser-vation**	**Question-naires**
Applicably in Phase	All	All	Design	Design	Final testing	All
Required Time	Low	Medium	High	High	Medium	Low
Needed Users	None	None	None	3+	20+	30+
Required Evaluators	3+	3+	1-2	1	1+	1
Required Equipment	Low	Low	Low	High	Medium	Low
Required Expertise	Medium	High	High	Medium	High	Low
Intrusive	No	No	No	Yes	Yes	No

Furthermore, as far as software usability is concerned, there are a number of different platforms on which software applications can be designed, developed, and evaluated. One of the most dominant platforms in today's computing environment is the Web. In the next section, the importance of the Web and methods commonly used to evaluate Web sites will be discussed.

2.5   Usability Evaluation of Web Sites

It is generally accepted that the development of the Internet has changed the face of digital computing forever, and Internet technologies have introduced many changes in the way people interact with computers too. The days of stand-alone PCs have almost disappeared; almost every computer user today knows how to go online. Besides, the Internet is so intriguing that many people are spending more time using the Internet but less time with family and friends (O'Toole, 2000).

Among the various applications of the Internet, the Web and E-mail are by far the most popular, outrunning other Internet services such as Telnet and FTP (File Transfer Protocol). So what exactly is the Web? Mayhew (1998, p. 1) provides us with a clear definition of the Web as follows:

> It is a huge, ever-growing collection of hyperlinked documents created by independent authors, stored on computers known as Web servers, and made accessible to anyone over

the Internet via software applications called browsers and various search engines accessible through browsers. Browsers provide a relatively user-friendly interface (at least compared to trying to use the Internet in the days before browsers) for navigating and viewing the total information space represented by all sites on the WWW. Thus, whereas the Internet is an electronic communications network that generally supports various kinds of communications including E-mail, the WWW represents a repository of public information created by the public and accessible to the public via the Internet.

Because of the easy-to-use graphical user interface in most Web browsers, the Web has been able to replace numerous text-based Internet services that used to receive significant attention but now hardly anybody knows, including Veronica, Archie, and WAIS (Wide Area Information Service). Thanks to the Web, various kinds of information are now available faster and more freely than ever before, in the form of Web pages to which everyone can gain access. However, accessible does not always mean usable. There are still many Web sites with bad design and poor navigation, which make them difficult to use. Web sites with poor usability can lead to various negative effects as pointed out by Borges, Morales, and Rodriguez (1998, p. 137):

- Users are frustrated, because of an inability to find the information sought, disorganized pages and confusing information, pages under construction and disconnected links, the lack of navigation support, and other problems.
- Exploration is discouraged, because of barriers imposed by the poorly designed interface and users' lack of trust or faith in the site.
- Time is wasted, because of disorganized pages, misleading link names, long pages, and long download times.
- Internet traffic is increased, because the problems just mentioned not only affect the use of a particular site, but are also responsible for much unnecessary traffic on the Internet.

These are reasons the evaluation of Web usability is a very important topic. Web site evaluation is also important to Web site owners because it is not cost-effective to publish Web sites that few people can use. With some level of evaluation, Web site owners can be more confident that their Web sites will be accessible and usable by most users.

There are some differences between Web sites and application software. First, Web sites can be accessed by any computer regardless of the operating system on which it runs, provided that it has a suitable Web browser. On the other hand, application software needs to be developed specifically for one operating system or a set of compatible operating systems only. Second, for application software, most executions are processed on the user's computer. But in the case of Web sites, most of the processing is done on the server so the response time of a Web site is usually slower than that of application software. Third, and most important, contents available on Web sites and stand-alone software are usually different but they are not mutually exclusive; some applications might be suitable to run on the Web and also on a PC as stand-alone software, such as games, dictionaries, and encyclopedias. On the other hand, many kinds of application are strictly committed to run on bare operating systems only (not on Web browsers), such as word processing and spreadsheets.

However, because of the similarities between a Web site user interface and traditional software user interface, methods and techniques previously used to evaluate software usability can be adapted and used for the evaluation of Web sites as well. For example, the Cognitive Walkthrough for the Web (CWW) technique, based on the CoLiDes model (Kitajima, Blackmon, and Polson, 2000), has been proposed by Blackmon, Polson, Kitajima, and Lewis (2002, pp. 465-466) and contains the following steps:

1. Compiling a set of realistic user goals and intended selections
2. Using Latent Semantic Analysis (LSA) to estimate semantic similarity of goals, headings, and link labels
3. Identifying problematic heading/link labels
4. Finding goal-specific problems

In addition to cognitive walkthrough, heuristic evaluation can also be used for Web usability evaluation. For instance, Nielsen's (1994a) classic usability heuristics have been adapted by Instone (1997a) for the usability evaluation of Web sites. User surveys or questionnaires are also often used for Web site usability evaluation. Further discussion of heuristic evaluation and questionnaire for the Web will be found in Chapter 3. Since there are many usability heuristics available for Web usability evaluation, Turk (2000) has provided a useful contingent heuristic approach to select the most appropriate heuristics to be used for each Web site based on user characteristics and purpose of the Web site. Detailed information regarding the contingent heuristic approach will be discussed in Chapter 4.

Various guidelines are also available for Web usability evaluation; one good example is the Web site evaluation checklist provided by Gaffney (1998), which is reproduced in Appendix 2C.

The other usability evaluation method that was previously discussed in this chapter is the observation of user behaviour. This method is very useful and reliable because it involves real or prospective users, in contrast to other methods that depend mostly on expert's opinions (except for questionnaire). There are many techniques that we can use to observe users while they are using the Web; some of the prominent techniques are videotaping and event logging. One good example case study is discussed by Osterbauer, Kohle, Grechenig, and Tscheligi (2000) which uses videotaping combined with a questionnaire. There are also many tools available for Web usability evaluation using the event logging technique; one of them is the Web Event-logging Tool (WET) developed by Etgen and Cantor (1999). Another technique commonly used to evaluate Web sites via user testing is to ask users to find specific information on the Web site and use it to answer questions proposed by the evaluator. An example of such a test can be found in Corry, Frick, and Hansen (1997).

Various characteristics of users, such as age, gender, culture, and experience with the Web, often play an important role in their personal preferences, and therefore can also influence usability evaluations of Web sites. A recent study by Chadwick-Dias, McNulty, and Tullis (2003) shows that older users tend to have more difficulty using Web sites than younger users. Simon's (2001) research study also suggests that there are differences between cultural and gender-based perception and satisfaction with Web sites, in that the perceptions of Asians and

Latin/South Americans were found to be different from those of Europeans and North Americans, and female users within certain culture groups were found to have widely different preferences from their male counterparts. Users' Web experience can also impact their perceived usability of Web sites, as Piller and Miller (2001) discovered in their study that highly experienced users subjectively rated the most usable site (in their experiment) as the least usable.

2.6 Conclusion

At the beginning of this chapter, the importance of Human-Computer Interaction as a research field was discussed, and emphasis was made on usability evaluation. Various methods and techniques for Web site usability evaluation were also presented. According to the research study that forms this book, a contingent heuristic approach was utilised, together with eye gaze tracking, to compare the usability of multiple Web sites. These two techniques were chosen because they are relatively new compared to other techniques. Therefore, only a few research studies have been undertaken regarding these approaches. Although current literature shows that the two techniques can be implemented and used in the evaluation of Web site usability, more research studies which utilise these techniques in different contexts still need to be undertaken, in order to establish them as effective and efficient ways to evaluate Web sites. Hence the utilisation and evaluation of these two techniques were selected as part of this book.

The next chapter will discuss heuristic approaches towards Web usability evaluation in detail, as they are the important basis that the contingent heuristic approach builds upon, while the contingent heuristic approach itself and the eye gaze monitoring technique will be discussed in depth in Chapter 4 and Chapter 5, respectively.

3

Heuristic Approaches in
Web Usability Evaluation

3.1 Introduction

Chapter 2 discussed various usability evaluation methods and techniques, including heuristic approaches. Two main categories of heuristic approaches exist: *(1) heuristic evaluation (expert walkthrough)* and *(2) questionnaire (user survey)*. This chapter will discuss in more detail the definition of heuristics and how heuristics can be used for usability evaluation. The reason that heuristic technique is chosen for discussion here is not only because it was used as part of the research, but also because the heuristic technique is by far the most popular technique for usability evaluation. Thus it is important for usability evaluators to understand this technique and be able to utilise it when other techniques are not feasible or adequate.

Heuristics may be defined broadly as "general rules used to describe common properties of usable interfaces" (Nielsen, 1994a). However, since the inception of usability heuristics in the early 1990s, many aspects of user interface development have significantly changed. As is well known, one of the changes is that we have been moving from generic (all-in-one) user interfaces (e.g. DOS, UNIX) to specialised (task-specific) interfaces (e.g. Web browsers, word processors, games). This change is demanded by both users and developers. Most users feel more comfortable with specialised interfaces because they can learn how to use them easily. For example, one can quickly learn how to use a mobile phone, a handheld computer, and a portable audio player. However, if we combined these devices into one, the resulting product would be more complicated and difficult to use by many users. Of course, the benefit of space/cost-saving is present but can it outweigh the reduction in usability? Only the users can answer this question. From the developers' point of view, specialised user interfaces are also simpler and faster to develop than cramming too many features into one single interface.

Considering that there have always been changes in the development of user interfaces, the evaluation of user interfaces also has to change. Therefore, heuristics should be redefined as rules used to describe properties of usable interfaces, including general rules (applied to any user interface) and specific rules (applied to a specific type of user interface only). The degree of specification is open for usability evaluators to select. However, they have to remember that the more specific the rules, the more reliable the results. For example, some usability evaluators always use a common set of heuristics for all interfaces, including software applications and Web sites, while some evaluators use one set of heuristics to evaluate software applications and another set of heuristics to evaluate Web sites.

The Web has been growing rapidly over the past few years. Table 3.1 shows the number of Web sites over the last five years according to Zakon (2004).

Table 3.1   Number of Web sites during 1999-2003

Year	Number of Web Sites
1999	9,560,866
2000	25,675,581
2001	36,276,252
2002	35,543,105
2003	45,980,112

Because there are a large number of Web sites, it is not appropriate to evaluate all of them using the same set of heuristics, because some properties that seem to be suitable for one Web site might not be suitable for others. Therefore, recent research by Turk (2000, 2001) suggests that to evaluate a Web site, we should take into account the Web site's main purpose and characteristics of targeted users, in order to get suitable heuristics to be used for the evaluation of the Web site. This approach, called "the contingent heuristic approach," will be discussed further in the next chapter.

As mentioned earlier in this chapter, usability heuristics can be utilised via heuristic evaluation (expert walkthrough) or questionnaire. The next section discusses heuristic evaluation in detail.

3.2   Heuristic Evaluation

Jakob Nielsen, who is well-known for his support for heuristic evaluation, provides the definition of this technique as follows:

> Heuristic evaluation is the most popular of the usability inspection methods. Heuristic evaluation is done as a systematic inspection of a user interface design for usability. The goal of heuristic evaluation is to find the usability problems in the design so that they can

be attended to as part of an iterative design process. Heuristic evaluation involves having a small set of evaluators examine the interface and judge its compliance with recognized usability principles (the "heuristics"). (Nielsen, 2003)

Heuristic evaluation is usually chosen by usability evaluators as either the first or the last technique, depending on personal preference and the needs of the evaluation project. Many people choose heuristic evaluation first because it is less time-consuming and more cost-effective than other techniques, i.e. they see heuristic evaluation as a discount usability engineering technique. Using the discount usability engineering approach means that we do not have to use the "best" available technique because it might be too expensive or consume too much time, therefore most of the times just "good" is enough. Nielsen proposed three discount usability engineering techniques: scenarios, simplified thinking aloud, and heuristic evaluation (Nielsen, 1994b).

From Nielsen's definition, we can identify two important terms, which are at the heart of heuristic evaluation: *a small set of evaluators* (experts) and *recognised usability principles* (heuristics). A usability evaluation that involves these two factors is recognised as a heuristic evaluation. However, using one of them alone is not considered a proper form of heuristic evaluation (e.g. using heuristics without experts would be called using a "guidelines checklist"). The reason that experts are important for heuristic evaluation is because their experience counts. Some heuristics may seem simple and easy to check but most of them require an expert's experience to understand the underlying concepts. Therefore, although novice evaluators can conduct heuristic evaluation (e.g. depending on published heuristics), the results may not be as comprehensive and reliable as those from the evaluation done by experienced evaluators.

In addition, Kantner and Rosenbaum (1997) emphasise that three pieces of background information are also of great importance to the usability evaluator, especially when heuristic evaluation is performed: (1) the purpose of the Web site; (2) profiles of its intended users; and (3) typical scenarios for users accessing the site. Their applications for Web site usability evaluation are further elaborated as follows:

1. When discussing the purpose of a web site, it's helpful to consider three categories. Web sites that supply descriptions of companies (or other organizations) and their products, services, informational offerings, or events can be described as informational sites. Web sites that provide explicit links to extensive databases are called search sites. Web sites that behave like products, where users perform other tasks in addition to reading or retrieving information, are referred to as transactional sites. Multi-purpose sites blur these boundaries.
2. Unfortunately, the definition of user in our increasingly Web-centric environment is becoming more vague, because "anyone can access the site." However, we must keep in mind which site visitors are the most likely—or the most welcome—and focus usability efforts on those subgroups.
3. Finally, the scenario for accessing a web site might be a straightforward URL to a home page, or a more roundabout path through a link in search-engine results to a page deep in the bowels of a site. Evaluators should keep in mind that any web page might be the user's door to that web site. Although users may perform more complex tasks in transactional sites, the free-form nature of navigation in any type of web site makes

ensuring (and measuring) success more complex in the Web environment. (Kantner and Rosenbaum, 1997)

There are various sets of usability heuristics that experts may choose. The most popular is a set of ten usability heuristics by Nielsen (1994a). This set of heuristics can be applied to many platforms, including the Web. For example, Instone (1997a) provides an adaptation of Nielsen's usability heuristics that can be used for Web evaluation.

3.3 Conducting Heuristic Evaluation

Danino (2001) provided a step-by-step guide on how to conduct a heuristic evaluation for the Web, as follows:

Step 1: Plan Your Evaluation
How will you test your interface? Heuristic Evaluation typically employs one of the three main approaches:
1.   Develop a set of tasks and ask your evaluators to carry them out.
2.   Provide evaluators with the goals of the system, and allow them to develop their own tasks.
3.   Ask evaluators to assess your dialogue elements.
Choosing which method to use will depend on you, the time that you have available, and on your evaluators.

Step 2: Choose your Evaluators
The more evaluators you use, the more usability problems you'll reveal. However, studies on the subject have shown that the benefit/cost ratio decreases at about five evaluators. [...] Heuristic Evaluation is known to find more than 90% of usability problems if it's performed by 3 to 5 experienced people.

Step 3: Review the Heuristics
Once you've decided which approach you'll take, and you've selected your evaluators, you'll need to brief these people on the ten heuristics [assuming Nielsen's] you want them to assess your site against.

Step 4: Conducting the Evaluation
Conduct the evaluation using either of these methods:
*   Individual Evaluation - each evaluator reviews the interface individually and reports problems to you. Individual evaluation is easily conducted over the Internet. It will pick up more problems than group evaluation, but takes a lot more time to complete.
*   Group Evaluation - evaluators review the interface as a team, while you record the problems. Evaluators do not have to agree on a problem - but every issue they identify should be recorded. Group evaluation requires more planning than does individual evaluation, as all evaluators need to be assembled, however, the evaluation need only be conducted once as all the evaluators can complete their tasks at the same time.

Step 5: Analysing your Results
Once your evaluators have worked their way through the tasks or goals you set, evaluated each of these in light of the ten heuristics, and provided their feedback, you'll need to compile all the information. Remove any duplicates and combine similar issues. What's left will be a set of problems or comments that you can address to improve your site's usability.

Danino (2001) also suggested her own interpretation of Nielsen's usability heuristics for the Web, which is, in many ways, similar to Instone's (1997a). Xerox (1996) has also provided a process for performing a heuristic evaluation (Appendix 3A).

Even though there are ten usability heuristics (according to Nielsen's set of usability heuristics) that can be applied in the process of Web evaluation, there may be only some of them which are highly critical to a particular Web site, and thus deserve more attention than others. Therefore, the contingent heuristic approach, as discussed in the next chapter, can be helpful when a heuristic evaluation is conducted.

Once the usability heuristics (also called "dimensions" by Turk (2000, 2001)) to be used in the evaluation process are selected, experts then examine the Web site according to the selected heuristics/dimensions and develop a list of detailed problems and suggestions for redesigning the site. However, if there is more than one expert evaluating a Web site, they are likely to have different ideas and comments. This is desirable because more flaws can be uncovered in the Web site, but sometimes it can make the analysis more difficult. Therefore, it is also possible to give a common set of questions to the experts and ask all of them to answer those questions in addition to their own suggestions. For example, Instone (1997b) provided the following questions that experts should answer while conducting a heuristic evaluation:

Regarding user control:
- Can users override this feature?
- Can they customize to suit their tastes or needs?
- Will giving users control of this feature reduce the usability of the site?

Regarding structure:
- If a user were taken directly to this page from an outside site, what could they figure out about the rest of the site from this one page?
- Is the site "brand" present?
- Is it clear which part of the site they are in?
- Is it clear how to navigate to other parts of the site?

Regarding design for change:
- How is old content archived?
- How is new content added?
- Can this design withstand the addition of 20 times the current content?

Another example of usability heuristic questions is Naughton's (1995). This set of questions was intended to be used by experts to give quick feedback to the designer while the interface was still under construction, but it can also be used for the finished interface as well. A slightly shortened version of Naughton's heuristic questions can be found in Appendix 3B.

There are various formats that can be used to document heuristic evaluation. However, the most appropriate format is a collection of questions or statements with Likert scale answer choices and additional space for comments, as shown in Figure 3.1.

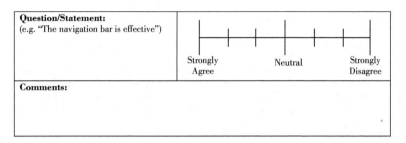

Question/Statement: (e.g. "The navigation bar is effective")	
	Strongly Agree Neutral Strongly Disagree
Comments:	

Figure 3.1   Heuristic evaluation documenting format

The questions and/or statements that should be included in a heuristic evaluation are usually dependent on the Web site to be evaluated. Different Web sites may be suitable for different sets of questions/statements. For example, according to Nielsen's usability heuristics, the questions in Table 3.2 which were selected (according to the Web site to be tested which, in this example, is a university Web site) from a comprehensive list of questions suggested by Brajnik (2003) may be asked.

Table 3.2 Sample questions for heuristic evaluation (Brajnik, 2003)

Visibility of system status	• Are important buttons/links visible without scrolling? • The page has a clear goal? • Is most important thing on the top of the page? • Is new content highlighted in home/base pages? • Can I understand that something is a link/button/control?
Match between system and the real world	• Appropriate labels are used for links/controls/categories/groupings? • Language is appropriate for audience? • Time information is present? • Are authors shown? Can I contact them?
User control and freedom	• Is a Flash introduction avoided? Can it be easily skipped? • Page has a "previous page" and "home" button? • Do these buttons work properly even from within framed pages? • Are breadcrumbs clearly shown? • Restrictions on browsers versions are shown and handled in some way?
Consistency and standards	• Anchor name is consistent with destination title? • Page title is consistent with page content? • Is same style, color, font used for similar objects in this page and throughout the site? • Page layout is consistent throughout the site? • Links colors are consistent with WWW conventions?
Error prevention	• Are navigation errors (dead-ends, loops, dangling pointers, getting lost) prevented from occurring? • Are unambiguous link descriptions/anchors used? • Do URLs use simple characters (avoiding non letters, long and complex names)? • In using forms, are error prevented (via menus, list of choices, ...)? • In using query mechanisms, are starting points available (suggesting general terms, or classification codes, ...)?
Recognition rather than recall	• Are links overwhelming (in number and layout)? • Is page content recognizable from link name? • Pictures do have meaningful captions? • Are links/controls clearly visible? • Clickable images are recognizable as such?
Flexibility and efficiency of use	• Can pages be bookmarked unambiguously? • Are search tools provided in the site? • Can people go into greater depth if they want? • Are pages written to be found (i.e. using HTML META information)?
Aesthetic and minimalist design	• Are buttons/links grouped according to function? • Are less important things (paragraphs, links, buttons) minimized? • Is the page succinct? • Are long list classified in chunks? • Are unneeded images, animations and blinkings avoided?
Help users recognize, diagnose, and recover from errors	• Are constructive suggestions provided for navigation errors? • Are natural explanations given of what happened and why?
Help and documentation	• How "far" is the help material (how well integrated and accessible from page)?

As an example, one question is selected from each heuristic category and used as a statement to conduct a heuristic evaluation of the Murdoch University home page[1] (Figure 3.2).

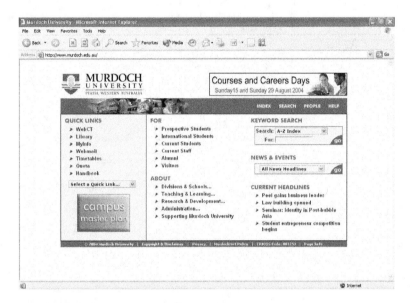

Figure 3.2 Murdoch University home page

Table 3.3 shows the heuristic evaluation of this Web page, which a usability expert may conduct.

---

[1] http://www.murdoch.edu.au

Table 3.3   Heuristic evaluation of Murdoch University home page by the author

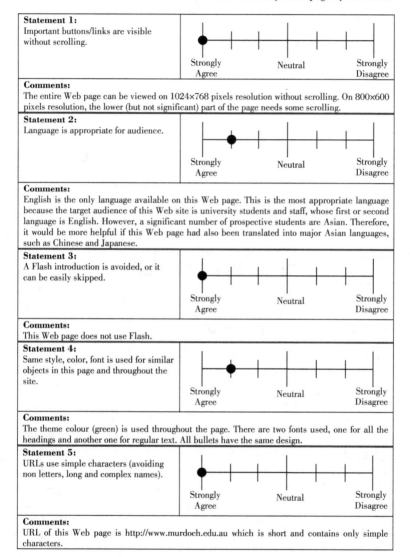

Statement 1: Important buttons/links are visible without scrolling.	*(Strongly Agree — Neutral — Strongly Disagree; marked at Strongly Agree)*

Comments:
The entire Web page can be viewed on 1024×768 pixels resolution without scrolling. On 800×600 pixels resolution, the lower (but not significant) part of the page needs some scrolling.

Statement 2: Language is appropriate for audience.	*(Strongly Agree — Neutral — Strongly Disagree; marked near Strongly Agree)*

Comments:
English is the only language available on this Web page. This is the most appropriate language because the target audience of this Web site is university students and staff, whose first or second language is English. However, a significant number of prospective students are Asian. Therefore, it would be more helpful if this Web page had also been translated into major Asian languages, such as Chinese and Japanese.

Statement 3: A Flash introduction is avoided, or it can be easily skipped.	*(Strongly Agree — Neutral — Strongly Disagree; marked at Strongly Agree)*

Comments:
This Web page does not use Flash.

Statement 4: Same style, color, font is used for similar objects in this page and throughout the site.	*(Strongly Agree — Neutral — Strongly Disagree; marked near Strongly Agree)*

Comments:
The theme colour (green) is used throughout the page. There are two fonts used, one for all the headings and another one for regular text. All bullets have the same design.

Statement 5: URLs use simple characters (avoiding non letters, long and complex names).	*(Strongly Agree — Neutral — Strongly Disagree; marked at Strongly Agree)*

Comments:
URL of this Web page is http://www.murdoch.edu.au which is short and contains only simple characters.

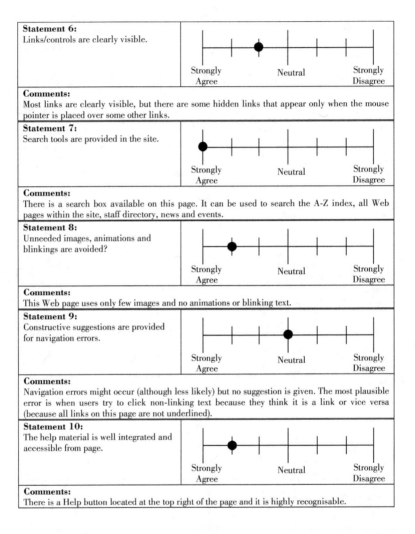

Statement 6: Links/controls are clearly visible.	Strongly Agree Neutral Strongly Disagree

Comments:
Most links are clearly visible, but there are some hidden links that appear only when the mouse pointer is placed over some other links.

Statement 7: Search tools are provided in the site.	Strongly Agree Neutral Strongly Disagree

Comments:
There is a search box available on this page. It can be used to search the A-Z index, all Web pages within the site, staff directory, news and events.

Statement 8: Unneeded images, animations and blinkings are avoided?	Strongly Agree Neutral Strongly Disagree

Comments:
This Web page uses only few images and no animations or blinking text.

Statement 9: Constructive suggestions are provided for navigation errors.	Strongly Agree Neutral Strongly Disagree

Comments:
Navigation errors might occur (although less likely) but no suggestion is given. The most plausible error is when users try to click non-linking text because they think it is a link or vice versa (because all links on this page are not underlined).

Statement 10: The help material is well integrated and accessible from page.	Strongly Agree Neutral Strongly Disagree

Comments:
There is a Help button located at the top right of the page and it is highly recognisable.

Even though heuristic evaluation is a powerful usability evaluation technique as it utilises the expertise of evaluators in evaluating Web sites against a set of rules (heuristics/dimensions), a high dependence on expert opinions can lead to prejudice, especially when only one expert is involved in the evaluation process. Furthermore, the validity of responses from surrogate users (acted by experts) is often questioned, as emphasised by the following quote:

Real users always surprise us: they often have problems we don't expect, and they sometimes breeze through where we expect them to bog down. Other reasons why heuristic evaluation shouldn't replace studying actual users are that it rarely emulates all the key audience groups for the site, and it doesn't necessarily indicate which problems users will encounter most frequently. (Kantner and Rosenbaum, 1997)

To overcome this problem, using a questionnaire is an alternative solution. A usability questionnaire also utilises usability heuristics like the heuristic evaluation does; however, it depends on user opinions rather than expert opinions.

3.4 Usability Questionnaire

Questionnaires and surveys exist as methods of evaluation because it makes sense that if we want to know how people think, we should ask them. Therefore, questionnaires and surveys have long been used in many fields of study, and information technology is no exception. If we want to evaluate the usability of a system, we should ask the users of that system. Questions to be asked can be yes/no questions, open-ended questions, multiple-choice questions, etc. However, the most popular type of questions for usability evaluation is Likert type questions as in the example in Table 3.3, i.e. users are given a statement and asked to rate their agreement with that statement. For example, three-point Likert scale can be *Disagree / Neutral / Agree*, or five-point Likert scale can be *Strongly Disagree / Disagree / Neutral / Agree / Strongly Agree.*

One prominent example of a questionnaire developed specifically for Web site usability evaluation is WAMMI (Website Analysis and MeasureMent Inventory). It was developed by the same people who developed SUMI (see Chapter 2), therefore it has many similar aspects to the SUMI questionnaire. For example, WAMMI is able to measure five usability factors, which are almost identical to those of SUMI:

1. Attractiveness: degree to which users like the site, whether they find the site pleasant to use.
2. Control: degree to which users feel 'in charge', whether the site allows them to navigate through it with ease, and whether the site communicates with them about what it is doing.
3. Efficiency: degree to which users feel that the site has the information they are looking for, that it works at a reasonable speed and is adapted to their browser.
4. Helpfulness: degree to which users feel that the site enables them to solve their problems with finding information and navigating.
5. Learnability: degree to which users feel they can get to use the site if they come into it for the first time, and the degree to which they feel they can learn to use other facilities or access other information once they have started using it. (Kirakowski, Claridge, and Whitehand, 1998)

The version of WAMMI that is available publicly is the basic version, which is composed of 20 questions, using a five-point Likert scale, in contrast to the commercial version which includes 60 questions. Details of the basic WAMMI questionnaire can be found in Table 3.4.

Table 3.4   Basic WAMMI questionnaire

Usability Question	Strongly agree	Agree	Undecided	Disagree	Strongly disagree
1. This web site has much that is of interest to me.	☐	☐	☐	☐	☐
2. It is difficult to move around this web site.	☐	☐	☐	☐	☐
3. I can quickly find what I want on this web site.	☐	☐	☐	☐	☐
4. This web site seems logical to me.	☐	☐	☐	☐	☐
5. This web site needs more introductory explanations.	☐	☐	☐	☐	☐
6. The pages on this web site are very attractive.	☐	☐	☐	☐	☐
7. I feel in control when I'm using this web site.	☐	☐	☐	☐	☐
8. This web site is too slow.	☐	☐	☐	☐	☐
9. This web site helps me find what I am looking for.	☐	☐	☐	☐	☐
10. Learning to find my way around this web site is a problem.	☐	☐	☐	☐	☐
11. I don't like using this web site.	☐	☐	☐	☐	☐
12. I can easily contact the people I want to on this web site.	☐	☐	☐	☐	☐
13. I feel efficient when I'm using this web site.	☐	☐	☐	☐	☐
14. It is difficult to tell if this web site has what I want.	☐	☐	☐	☐	☐
15. Using this web site for the first time is easy.	☐	☐	☐	☐	☐
16. This web site has some annoying features.	☐	☐	☐	☐	☐
17. Remembering where I am on this web site is difficult.	☐	☐	☐	☐	☐
18. Using this web site is a waste of time.	☐	☐	☐	☐	☐
19. I get what I expect when I click on things on this web site.	☐	☐	☐	☐	☐
20. Everything on this web site is easy to understand.	☐	☐	☐	☐	☐

Other than WAMMI, Tullis and Stetson (2004) suggest that the following questionnaires can also be used for Web site usability evaluation:

1. SUS (System Usability Scale)—This questionnaire, developed at Digital Equipment Corp., consists of ten questions. It was adapted by replacing the word "system" in every question with "website". Each question is a statement and a rating on a five-point scale of "Strongly Disagree" to "Strongly Agree".

2. QUIS (Questionnaire for User Interface Satisfaction)—The original questionnaire, developed at the University of Maryland, was composed of 27 questions. We dropped three that did not seem to be appropriate to websites (e.g., "Remembering names and use of commands"). The term "system" was replaced by "website", and the term "screen" was generally replaced by "web page". Each question is a rating on a ten-point scale with appropriate anchors at each end (e.g., "Overall Reaction to the Website: Terrible ... Wonderful").

3. CSUQ (Computer System Usability Questionnaire)—This questionnaire, developed at IBM, is composed of 19 questions. The term "system" or "computer system" was replaced by "website". Each question is a statement and a rating on a seven-point scale of "Strongly Disagree" to "Strongly Agree".

4. Words (adapted from Microsoft's Product Reaction Cards)—This questionnaire is based on the 118 words used by Microsoft on their Product Reaction Cards. Each word was presented with a check-box and the user was asked to choose the words that best

describe their interaction with the website. They were free to choose as many or as few words as they wished. (Tullis and Stetson, 2004)

WAMMI, as well as other questionnaires discussed above, is an example of a non-contingent tool, i.e. the same set of questions is used for every Web site evaluated. One major drawback of a non-contingent questionnaire is that we can ask only general questions (i.e. questions applicable to all Web sites) but we cannot ask specific questions because these questions may introduce bias to the results. Therefore, the feedback we gain from the users is limited. On the other hand, if we can ask specific questions that are different for each Web site, we can gain richer information from the users. This is the reason we need the contingent heuristic approach. The use of the contingent heuristic approach in Web usability evaluation will be discussed in more detail in the next chapter.

3.5   Conclusion

This chapter discussed heuristic-based approaches commonly used in Web usability evaluation, including heuristic evaluations and questionnaires. The definition and process of heuristic evaluation specifically for the Web have been discussed, together with some examples of usability heuristics and questions. A heuristic evaluation documentation of a real Web page was provided as an example. Finally, a usability questionnaire was discussed as an alternative technique to heuristic evaluation. The advantages of questionnaire were discussed, as well as an example of a Web usability questionnaire.

4

Contingent Heuristic Approach for Web Usability Evaluation

4.1 Introduction

In this chapter, the contingent heuristic approach for Web usability evaluation as proposed by Turk (2000, 2001) will be discussed. The contingent heuristic approach is useful because it can be applied to various usability evaluation methods, especially heuristic evaluation and questionnaires. It can be clarified that the usability of a particular system is contingent upon its users, tasks, and context of use. In the case of Web sites, context of use would include bandwidth of the connection, browser type, hardware used, etc. Therefore, usability evaluators should consider these factors and select only criteria that are applicable to their users, tasks, and context, rather than using all available criteria. For example, not all of the 60 questions in the WAMMI questionnaire may be of importance to a particular Web site user or task, so it is appropriate to delete some unrelated questions and select only a subset of them. Furthermore, it is also beneficial to the response rate of the survey because, as the questionnaire gets shorter, users feel less frustrated and are more likely to complete it. Evidence for this assumption was provided in Kalantar and Talley's (1999) research study which demonstrated that the response rates for their health survey were higher among those receiving the short, rather than the long, questionnaire. The same is true for online (Web-based) surveys. Nielsen (2004) suggests that the number of questions in an online survey be kept to a minimum and only relevant questions be asked.

At present there are a considerable number of non-contingent Web usability evaluation tools readily available on the market. These non-contingent tools (available in the form of usability heuristics or questionnaire) are usually provided with very little or no capacity for customisation. Therefore, by adopting these tools, evaluators often use all of the heuristics or questions included in the package; otherwise they can select relevant criteria manually. However, without a formal approach, manual selection tends to be subjective and unpredictable. Therefore, Turk (2001) emphasises the importance of the contingent heuristic approach, as follows:

> If one is to carry out the most effective heuristic evaluation for a particular WWW site it is necessary to choose the most relevant set of criteria from the vast array available. It is also important to establish a priority order for the criteria, since specific pairs of criteria (guidelines) may be contradictory. Also, there are too many criteria for them all to be practically used in any particular evaluation procedure. Following the 'user-centred' and 'task-based' paradigm of HCI, the selection of heuristic evaluation criteria should be based on the characteristics of the target user group and the site purpose – i.e. a 'contingent' approach.

Defining user characteristics and Web site purpose as two main indicators involved in the criteria selection process, Turk (2001) further classifies user characteristics and Web site purpose as follows:

User characteristics:
    A. Age
    B. Culture
    C. Disabilities
    D. Education level
    E. WWW/IT Experience
Categories of WWW site purpose:
    I. Communication (e-mail; discussion lists; chat groups)
    II. Information (e.g. educational material; news)
    III. Entertainment (e.g. games; gambling; pornography)
    IV. Services (e.g. search engines; software libraries; counselling)
    V. Electronic Commerce / marketing (business-customer and business-business)

Other characteristics of the users (e.g. gender, location, interests, etc.) can also be appended to the above list depending on their applicability to the Web site.

4.2 Website Usability Contingent Evaluation Tool (WUCET)

In addition to providing the conceptual framework for the contingent heuristic approach, Turk (2001) has also suggested a systematic way to carry out the contingent heuristic approach by introducing the contingency table, which represents the relationship between user characteristics, Web site purpose, and usability dimensions. One possible format of the contingency table, suggested by Turk, is shown in Table 4.1.

Table 4.1 Section of the contingency table (Turk, 2001)

			Usability Dimension*					
			1. Content	2. Hyperlinks	3. Clarity/ Presentation	4. Adherence to Conventions/ Standards	5. Navigation Support	6. Search Facilities
User Characteristics	A. Age	Young						
		Middle-Aged						
		Old	A[1]	A[2]	A[3]	A[4]	A[5]	A[6]
		General						
	B. Culture	Western	B[1]	B[2]	B[3]	B[4]	B[5]	B[6]
		Asian						
		General						
	C. Disabilities	Visual						
		Hearing	C[1]	C[2]	C[3]	C[4]	C[5]	C[6]
		Cognitive						
		None						
	D. Education Level	Primary						
		Secondary						
		Tertiary/Post						
		General	D[1]	D[2]	D[3]	D[4]	D[5]	D[6]
	E. Web/IT Experience	Low						
		High						
		General	E[1]	E[2]	E[3]	E[4]	E[5]	E[6]
	Average		AVG[1]	AVG[2]	AVG[3]	AVG[4]	AVG[5]	AVG[6]
Web Site Purpose	I. Communication							
	II. Information							
	III. Entertainment							
	IV. Services							
	V. E-Commerce/Marketing		W[1]	W[2]	W[3]	W[4]	W[5]	W[6]
	Final Product		PROD[1]	PROD[2]	PROD[3]	PROD[4]	PROD[5]	PROD[6]

* The full table consists of 16 usability dimensions (listed in Table 4.2)

A comprehensive list of Web usability dimensions/criteria was also provided by Turk (2000, 2001) as shown in Table 4.2.

Table 4.2   Usability dimensions (Turk, 2000; 2001)

a)	Content: usefulness; relevance; accuracy; truthfulness; completeness; currency
b)	Hyperlinks: quantity; quality; relevance; currency (dangling?)
c)	Clarity / Presentation: simplicity; elegance; layout structure; use of graphics; readability
d)	Adherence to Conventions/Standards: to the extent that they apply to the site purpose
e)	Navigation Support: structured layout; site map; navigation buttons; search; links; frames
f)	Search Facilities: functionality; utility
g)	Attractiveness / Annoyance: images; video; sounds; animations; banners; creativity; innovations
h)	Interaction Opportunities: creativity; functionality; utility
i)	Error Reduction / Recovery: design to limit errors; undo facility
j)	Help / Documentation: availability; utility
k)	Download Speed: number and format of graphics; thumbnails; progressive build up
l)	H/W and S/W[1] Requirements: restrictions; reliance on downloads; needing latest browser version
m)	Reliability: does server go down often
n)	Customisability: user model / profile; cookies for user attributes
o)	Ease of Downloads: range of material available; formats of files
p)	Integrity / Ethics: security (e.g. use of credit card no / email address); race / gender treatment

Apart from the format of the contingency table and the list of usability dimensions, the contents of the table cells are also equally important (if not more so). Turk (2001) has suggested some of the relationships that should be represented in the contingency table in Table 4.3. Some of these relationships can be inferred from first principles and others will need to be established by relevant review of literature or by research studies.

---

[1] Hardware and Software

Table 4.3   Suggested relationships in the contingency table (Turk, 2001)

Regarding User Characteristics
• Younger users will be more concerned with site Attractiveness (dimension 'g') than Reliability (m)
• Users from non-western cultures may see Customisability (n) as a high priority
• The top priority for visually impaired users will be Clarity of Presentation (c)
• The quality of Content (a) may be the top priority of users with high education levels, while for those with low education, the availability of Help/Documentation (j) may be more important
• Users with high WWW/IT experience will be more concerned about Search Facilities (f) and Interaction Opportunities (h) than with Error Reduction/Recovery (i)
Regarding WWW Site Purpose
• For sites where communication is the main purpose, Download Speed (k) and H/W / S/W Requirements (l) may be critical issues
• For informational sites Hyperlinks (b), Navigation Support (e), Search Facilities (f) and Download Speed (k) are priorities
• The top priority for entertainment sites is probably Attractiveness (g), followed by Interaction Opportunities (h) and Download Speed (k)
• For services sites, Download Speed (k), Reliability (m) and Ease of Download (o) are critical dimensions
• For e-commerce sites, Adherence to Conventions/Standards (d) and Navigational Support (e) are important, as well as Attractiveness (g) and Integrity/Ethics(p)

Once the contingency table is fully developed (i.e. each cell is filled with a priority value, which is a number ranging from 1.0 to 5.0 according to its priority), the analysis is straightforward. The evaluator selects user characteristics and a Web site purpose that match the Web site being evaluated. For example, suppose that we are evaluating an electronic commerce Web site selling hearing aids. The company that owns this Web site is based in the U.S.A., and this company does not ship products outside the U.S.A. due to the potential for credit card fraud. Therefore, the primary users of this Web site are senior American citizens with hearing impairment. Using this information, we highlight the rows of related user characteristics and Web site purpose as shown in Table 4.1. Then for each usability dimension, we calculate the average of the priority value of each selected user characteristic $\{AVG[i] = (A[i] + B[i] + C[i] + D[i] + E[i]) \div 5; i = 1...16\}$ and multiply it with the priority value of the selected Web site purpose to yield the final product $\{PROD[i] = AVG[i] \times W[i]\}$. These final products represent the importance of each usability dimension as applied to the users and the purpose of the Web site to be evaluated. The higher the number, the more important the dimension is during usability evaluation and hence, the more important it is to include questions related to that dimension in an evaluation questionnaire.

    The example above is overly simplified, so the analysis can be done by creating a simple spreadsheet. However, as the number of usability dimensions and user characteristics increases, the need for automated tools arises. Furthermore, we might want to assign different weights to each user characteristic (the example above assumes equal weight) and that can make calculations too complicated to be done manually. Therefore, the contingency table was developed by Turk (2000, 2001) and the automated tool named WUCET (Website Usability Contingent Evaluation Tool) was developed by Dunstan (2003) in collaboration with Turk. The current version of the contingency table (which is also used in this study) can be found in Appendix 4A.

Since WUCET was developed as a software application based on the Microsoft Access platform, it can be run on many versions of Microsoft Windows operating system (e.g. Windows 2000, Windows XP) with Microsoft Access installed. The use of WUCET for usability evaluation is simple. First, the evaluator submits the intended user characteristics and the primary purpose of the Web site. Table 4.4 depicts options available for selection within the tool.

Table 4.4   WUCET options

Intended User Characteristics					Primary Web Site Purpose
Age	**Culture**	**Disabilities**	**Education**	**Web/IT Experience**	
General	General	None	General	General	Entertainment
Young	Asian	Cognitive	Primary	Low	Communication
Middle-Aged	Western	Hearing	Secondary	High	Information
Old		Visual	Tertiary/Post		Services
					E-Commerce
					Marketing

After the submission of user characteristics and site purpose, WUCET will generate a score of importance for each usability dimension for that Web site. The higher the score, the more important the usability dimension is to the Web site. In addition to the scores, WUCET also provides a recommended set of questions that the evaluator can use to conduct a usability survey with his/her Web site visitors. There are 20 questions provided for each Web site (except in some special cases, which will be discussed later) which WUCET selects from the built-in question pool. The question pool consists of three questions per usability dimension (see Appendix 4B). According to the scores, WUCET selects three questions for each of the top three ranked dimensions, two questions for each of the next three ranked dimensions, and one question for each of the next five ranked dimensions. However, in the case where there is a tie between the third and the fourth dimensions, between the sixth and the seventh dimensions, or between the eleventh and the twelfth dimensions, one more question might be added, so the total number of questions can be 21.

Dunstan (2003) also conducted a comparative study between the contingent heuristic approach represented by WUCET (his own development) and the non-contingent heuristic approach represented by WAMMI (Website Analysis and MeasureMent Inventory) developed by Kirakowski and Cierlik (1998). In his research study, he proposed the following two hypotheses:

H1: A contingency-based approach to WWW site usability evaluation can be successfully implemented via a spreadsheet-based tool (WUCET)

H2: A contingency-based WWW site usability evaluation tool (WUCET) will be more effective than a non-contingency based one (WAMMI) (Dunstan, 2003, p. 48)

In order to test these hypotheses, he developed the contingency-based Web site usability evaluation tool (WUCET) by using a commercially available spreadsheet development software. The main component of WUCET is the contingency table, which is based on the work of Turk (2001) as discussed earlier in this section. The primary reasons that he chose to represent the contingency table in spreadsheet form were:

1. Usability dimensions can be represented within 'cells', where they can contain a relevant values or formulas.
2. These values and formulas can be referenced according to specific usability dimensions/criteria in a matrix format.
3. Recalculations are possible according to cell formulas and differing values. (Dunstan, 2003, p. 58)

Dunstan also suggested possible inputs, outputs, and calculations of WUCET as shown in Table 4.5.

Table 4.5   Inputs, outputs, and calculations for WUCET (Dunstan, 2003, p. 61)

Inputs	Outputs
• Website Purpose (Dominant) • User Characteristics (Dominant)	• Overall Priority Rating for Usability (dimensions a–p) • List of the most effective set of dimensions (criteria) • One or more questions (automated questionnaire) for each usability dimension, based on the priority rating
Calculations	
For each instance of Website Purpose and User Characteristics: Dimension (a-p) Rating = Product of the Mean Rating Value of User Characteristics (A-E) and Dominant Purpose (I-V)	

Two laboratory experiments were conducted to gather data for hypothesis testing. In the first experiment (Experiment A), there were 67 respondents, all of whom were university students. Each participant was asked to view three Web sites and answer two separate questionnaires for each Web site, one generated by WUCET and the other generated by a simulated version of WAMMI (as the researcher did not have access to the commercial version). After the evaluation of the Web sites, respondents also evaluated the evaluative process itself (meta-evaluation) by answering some qualitative questions. A few months later, a second experiment (Experiment B) was conducted in the same fashion as Experiment A, in order to confirm the findings from Experiment A. However, some technical aspects of WUCET (e.g. user interface, processing speed, etc.) were revised based on feedback from Experiment A, to make it more effective and more efficient. Experiment B utilised a different set of respondents to Experiment A. There were 35 respondents in Experiment B, and they were also university students.

In order to test the first hypothesis (H1), qualitative data from the meta-evaluation was analysed and it was found that this hypothesis was supported by most respondents as they reported positive feedback regarding the WUCET tool utilised in the experiments with a high level of consistency.

The second hypothesis (H2) is more complex, therefore both quantitative and qualitative measures were used. First, a number of statistical tests were performed, including paired t-tests, which compared WUCET and WAMMI results for each Web site and each usability dimension. However, since both tools utilised different usability dimensions, a mapping between WAMMI and WUCET dimensions was necessary, as shown in Table 4.6.

Table 4.6   WAMMI and WUCET dimension comparison (Dunstan, 2003, p. 114)

WAMMI dimensions	WUCET dimensions
Attractiveness	Clarity / Presentation
	Attractiveness / Annoyance
Control	Hyperlinks
	Navigation Support
Efficiency	Content
	Search Facilities
	Interaction Opportunities
	Download Speed
	H/W and S/W Requirements
	Reliability
	Ease of Downloads
Helpfulness	Error Reduction / Recovery
	Help / Documentation
Learnability	Adherence to Conventions/Standards
	Customisability
Other	Integrity / Ethics

It was discovered from statistical tests that there was a significant difference in some usability dimensions between WUCET and WAMMI. Therefore, a further qualitative analysis was made to determine if WUCET is indeed more effective than WAMMI (to test the second hypothesis, H2). Again, qualitative data from the meta-evaluation, plus more elaborate responses obtained from the respondents after the experiments, was analysed and it was found that respondents preferred WUCET to WAMMI. Therefore, the second hypothesis was supported.

4.3   Web Usability Dimensions

As discussed earlier, the role of the contingent heuristic approach in Web usability evaluation is to help evaluators concentrate on the usability dimensions or criteria that are significantly related to their users and Web purpose. Apart from the work of Turk (2000, 2001), there are various other sets of Web usability dimensions/criteria that Web evaluators can choose. For example, Hassan and Li (2001) conducted a research study about Web usability criteria by analysing current literature on Web design/development and classifying these criteria into seven main categories (some with subcategories) as shown in Table 4.7.

Table 4.7   Categories of usability criteria (Hassan and Li, 2001)

Category	Subcategory
1. Screen design	a. Space allocation b. Choice of colour c. Readability d. Scannability
2. Content	a. Scope b. Accuracy c. Authority d. Currency e. Uniqueness f. Linkages
3. Accessibility	a. Loading speed b. Browser compatibility c. Search facility d. Web site accessibility
4. Navigation	-
5. Media use	a. Audio b. Graphics and images c. Animation and video
6. Interactivity	-
7. Consistency	-

Detailed information about criteria that fall into each of these categories can be found in Hassan and Li (2001) and is also reproduced in Appendix 4C.

Turk's (2000, 2001) and Hassan and Li's (2001) Web usability dimensions/criteria have many items in common: screen design (clarity/presentation), content, accessibility (search facilities, download speed, H/W and S/W requirements), navigation, media use (attractive/annoyance), and interactivity. However, there are quite a few differences. Turk takes into account error reduction/recovery and help/documentation while Hassan and Li do not have them on their list. These two dimensions are important because they are frequently needed by users. Another difference is that Turk focuses on adherence to conventions/standards (inter-site consistency), while Hassan and Li focuses on consistency within one's own Web site (intra-site consistency).

In addition to the usability dimensions/criteria already discussed, the following dimensions/criteria can also be used in the evaluation of Web sites:

- Steps or Web page depth to complete tasks (e.g. from adding products to the shopping cart to submitting payment)
- Openness or concealment (e.g. encrypted URLs, disabled view-source, disabled right-click)

- Response to users
    - Web page response (e.g. "You have been unsubscribed." vs. "We regret that you have chosen to unsubscribe. We respect your decision; however, if you would like to tell us how we could improve our service to win you back, please feel free to contact us. And of course, you are always welcome to re-subscribe at any time you wish. We look forward to your return.")
    - E-mail response (e.g. confirmation of order, tracking number)
- Follow-up contact with users (e.g. e-mails, newsletters, updates)
- Localisation (e.g. date/time format, multilinguality)
- Update frequency (e.g. every week, every month, never)
- Point of contact (e.g. live support, e-mail, feedback form)
- Accessibility (especially for people with disabilities), which is an important topic, as it is often confused with usability. However, accessibility and usability are two different things. Accessibility of a Web site means that all people, regardless of their disability, must be able to access and use the Web site without any difficulty. We can see that accessibility is closely related to usability; however, their foci are different. Usability focuses on a small target group of users but tries to maximise their satisfaction. On the other hand, accessibility ensures that a large variety of people can access a Web site with less concern about their satisfaction with it. Besides, usability always implies accessibility for target users but not vice versa (i.e. accessibility does not imply usability). In other words, in order for a Web site to be usable, it has to be accessible by target users. Therefore, accessibility evaluation has to be integrated as part of usability evaluation. Accessibility for non-disabled people is usually assessed by hardware/software requirements. However, for people with disabilities, accessibility requires more complicated analysis. Therefore, Web accessibility is not discussed in detail here, but more information can be found on the W3C Web site[2].

Once usability evaluators have selected specific Web usability dimensions to be used in the evaluation process, whether by manual selection or with the help of a contingency table, the next step is to choose usability evaluation methods and techniques suitable for each of the selected dimensions, as shown in Table 4.8.

---

[2] http://www.w3.org/WAI/

Table 4.8   Usability evaluation methods and techniques according to usability dimensions

Usability Dimension	Usability Evaluation Method / Technique
Content	Heuristic evaluation / Questionnaire
Hyperlinks	Web link validation Event logging
Clarity / Presentation	Heuristic evaluation / Questionnaire Guidelines User testing
Adherence to Conventions / Standards	Guidelines
Navigation Support	Expert walkthrough Cognitive walkthrough User testing
Search Facilities	User testing
Attractiveness / Annoyance	Heuristic evaluation / Questionnaire Guidelines User testing
Interaction Opportunities	Expert walkthrough User testing
Error Reduction / Recovery	Cognitive walkthrough User testing Event logging
Help / Documentation	Heuristic evaluation / Questionnaire
Download Speed	Guidelines Event logging
H/W and S/W Requirements	Guidelines
Reliability	Event logging
Customisability	Heuristic evaluation / Questionnaire
Ease of Downloads	Heuristic evaluation / Questionnaire Guidelines
Integrity / Ethics	Heuristic evaluation / Questionnaire Guidelines
Steps or Web page depth to complete tasks	Expert walkthrough Event logging
Openness / Concealment	Guidelines
Response to users	Heuristic evaluation / Questionnaire
Follow-up contact with users	Heuristic evaluation / Questionnaire
Localisation	Guidelines
Update frequency	Event logging
Point of contact	Heuristic evaluation / Questionnaire Guidelines
Accessibility	Heuristic evaluation / Questionnaire Guidelines User testing

From Table 4.8, we can see that many dimensions can be evaluated by heuristic evaluation or questionnaire. Therefore, if it is not feasible to combine various usability evaluation methods (especially when only one or a few Web sites are being evaluated), heuristic evaluation or questionnaire alone can be used as a substitute for other methods and still produce good results. For example, if there is no automated tool available for measuring the exact download speed of a Web site, we can still use a questionnaire to ask users what they think about the download speed or, in the case where heuristic evaluation is employed, get feedback about download speed from an expert.

4.4 Conclusion

In this chapter, the role of the contingent heuristic approach in Web usability evaluation has been discussed, including an introduction to the contingency table and the Website Usability Contingent Evaluation Tool (WUCET). Various Web usability dimensions that can be selected and used in the evaluation process have also been listed.

5

Eye Gaze Tracking for
Web Usability Evaluation

5.1   Introduction

As mentioned in Chapter 2, there are various methods and techniques that
can be used in the usability evaluation process. However, user testing is
considerably more effective than any other method because it is an empirical
method based on actual users doing actual tasks. User behaviour while performing a
test can be observed by different techniques, such as videotaping, thinking aloud,
event logging, and more recently, eye gaze tracking. It is generally accepted that
videotaping has been widely used because it is a non-intrusive way to observe users,
but it is difficult and time-consuming to do the analysis (i.e. to transform visual cues
into statistical data). Sometimes the videotaping technique is combined with
thinking aloud so that both user action and voice could be recorded and played back
by the observer. However, thinking aloud is often found intrusive and unnatural by
most users. On the other hand, the event logging technique, such as keystroke
recording and mouse movement/click monitoring is non-intrusive and generates
statistical data automatically, but it concentrates only on feedback from specific
physical interaction activities by users and overlooks the human perception process
and cognitive processing aspects. In contrast, the eye tracking technique uses
human eye perception as the main indicator of the interaction. Hence it has
advantages over the event logging techniques. Furthermore, it can also be used to
complement other data collection techniques.

One of the major benefits of the eye tracking method is that it can answer
various questions that traditional observation techniques cannot answer, as can be
seen in the following scenario provided by Karn, Ellis, and Juliano (2000):

Imagine, for example, that we observe users spending longer than expected looking at a particular software application window or a web page without making the appropriate selection to reach their goal. After situations such as these, participants often have difficulty reconstructing their thought pattern after the task or even verbalizing their thought processes in a "think aloud" protocol during the task. The experimenter has no idea what went wrong. Is it because the user overlooked the appropriate control or hyperlink? Did another visual element in the interface – perhaps an animated graphic – distract the user? Did users see the control, but fail to comprehend its meaning? Did they look at the corporate branding elements? [...] Without knowing the answers to these questions, design recommendations have to be implemented by trial and error, adding to development time and cost. Recording the movements of participants' eyes during task performance can offer additional information that may help us answer these kinds of questions and reduce trial and error in user interaction design.

Eye tracking is non-intrusive (with some technologies) and can provide statistical data promptly. It is considered one of the most promising techniques for observing users, and it was also used in the research that forms part of this book. Therefore, the eye tracking technique is discussed in depth in this chapter.

So what is eye tracking? EyeTracking, Inc. (2004) provides an overview of eye tracking as follows:

Eye-tracking is a technique used to determine where a person is looking. The concepts underlying eye-tracking are deceptively simple: track the movements of the user's eyes and note what the pupils are doing while the user is looking at a particular feature. In practice, however, these measures are difficult to achieve and require high-precision instruments as well as sophisticated data analysis and interpretation.

Renshaw, Finlay, Ward, and Tyfa (2002) provided an overview of progress in eye tracking research as follows:

Eye tracking in Human Computer Interaction is now moving into a more mature phase. Studies have established its potential both as a means of measuring usability and for controlling aspects of the human computer interface. The technology has progressed steadily from highly invasive procedures involving the attachment of eye caps to the cornea using anaesthetics to remote non-invasive tracking methods that do not involve any contact between the equipment and the participant. The only requirement is that the head is kept reasonably still. In addition, there have been developments in software that have both improved the control of eye tracking equipment and facilitated the analysis and visualisation of the large volumes of data produced. Assessing usability is increasingly important as interaction with computers becomes ubiquitous. Usability is enhanced by good design and eye tracking can make a contribution to a quantitative evaluation of how usable a particular design is.

Some frequently used eye tracking terms that will appear later in this chapter can also be found in Appendix 5A with their extended definitions.

5.2 Eye Tracking Tools: Hardware and Software

Since their introduction, eye tracking hardware and software tools have been used in the field of human-computer interaction primarily for two purposes (EyeTech Digital Systems, 2003):

1. To provide input from the user to the computer (run as "foreground"). In this mode, users interact with computers using their eyes; they can move the cursor around the screen, perform a selection, or type characters just by moving their eyes and sometimes by staring at specific points on the screen or blinking.

2. To observe user's eye movement characteristics (run as "background"). In this mode, users interact with computers in traditional ways (using mouse, keyboard, etc.); the eye tracker works in the background (invisible to the user, ideally) to gather data about eye movements of the user and later present it to the usability evaluator.

There are many eye tracking tools available at present. Since using eye tracking as an input device (foreground mode) is not the topic of discussion in this research, only eye tracking tools that support user observation (background mode) will be presented in this chapter.

Eye tracking tools can utilise various technologies for the eye gaze tracking process. These technologies usually fall into one of the following categories:

1. Electrode recording: One of the least expensive and simplest eye tracking technologies is recording from skin electrodes, like those used for making ECG[1] or EEG[2] measurements. Because the retina is electrically active compared to the rest of the eyeball, there is a measurable potential difference between it and the cornea. Electrodes are placed on the skin around the eye socket, and can measure changes in the orientation of this potential difference. However, this method is more useful for measuring relative eye movements than absolute position. It can cover a wider range of movement than other tracking technologies, but gives poor accuracy.

2. Contact lenses: The most accurate, but least user-friendly technology uses a physical attachment to the front of the eye. A non-slipping contact lens is ground to fit precisely over the corneal bulge, and then slight suction is applied (mechanically or chemically) to hold the lens in place. Once the contact lens is attached, the eye tracking problem reduces to tracking something affixed to the lens, and a variety of means can be used. This method is obviously practical only for laboratory studies, as it is very uncomfortable.

3. Remote camera: Most practical eye tracking methods are based on a noncontacting camera that observes the eyeball, plus image processing techniques to interpret the picture. The position of the eyeball can be identified by tracking one of its visible features. For example, the boundary between the sclera (white portion of the front of the eye) and iris (colored portion) is easy to find. (Corno, Farinetti, and Signorile, 2002)

Because eye tracking via electrode recording has poor accuracy and contact lenses are uncomfortable for the users, remote camera recording of eye gaze has gained the

---

[1] Electrocardiogram

[2] Electroencephalogram

most popularity, especially for usability research (Corno et al., 2002). The following is a summary of remote eye gaze tracking tools available on the market.

LC Technologies (2002) offers the Eyegaze Development System, which is available in both desktop and portable versions. The user's eye gaze behaviour is monitored by a camera attached to the computer monitor. For this system to work accurately, users are allowed to move their heads within a 3.8 cm range only. The double computer configuration is possible so that eye gaze data can be sent from the user's computer to the observer's computer via Ethernet LAN. The complete Eyegaze Development System contains hardware (PC, camera, etc.) and software development tool kit for calibration, demonstration, and data analysis.

Eye Response Technologies (2003) has developed the ERICA (Eye-gaze Response Interface Computer Aid) system, which combines hardware and software suitable for eye tracking research. The system is non-intrusive to the user because it uses a camera attached below the monitor. The ERICA system includes GazeTracker software, which is used to capture and analyse the user's eye gaze behaviour. According to Applied Science Laboratories (2003), GazeTracker serves three functions:

1. Stimulus Presentation: study eye response to still images, videos, or computer software, such as web content
2. Information Gathering: record all eye-tracking, mouse, and keyboard data in one place
3. Data Analysis and Visualization: easily view your data and output statistics based on user definable regions of interest and fixation data

In addition, GazeTracker offers many useful features for Web page analysis, including compensation for Web page scrolling and automatic generation of LookZones (possible regions of interest) by parsing the HTML source code of the page (Lankford, 2000).

Applied Science Laboratories (2003), which is also the sole distributor of ERICA's GazeTracker software, offers various eye tracking hardware and software systems. Regarding the hardware, many models are available, including model 501 (head-mounted) and model 504 (desk-mounted). These eye trackers come with operating software (EYEPOS) and data analysis software (EYENAL and FIXPLOT). Applied Science Laboratories also offers a system that combines eye tracking and head tracking (provided by Ascension Technology), so that the movement of the user's head does not affect the accuracy of eye tracking.

EyeTech Digital Systems (2003) offers the Quick Glance eye tracking system. There are two major versions: *Quick Glance 1* and *Quick Glance 2*, as shown in Table 5.1.

Table 5.1   Quick Glance eye tracking system comparisons

	Quick Glance 1	Quick Glance 2B	Quick Glance 2S	Quick Glance 2SH
Portability	Desktop Only	Desktop/Laptop	Desktop/Laptop	Desktop/Laptop
Connection to PC	Internal PCI card	1394 Port	1394 Port	1394 Port
Head Movement	4 by 4 cm	6 by 6 cm	6 by 6 cm	10 by 10 cm
Motion Tolerance*	2	3	4	4
Lighting Tolerance*	2	2	4	4
Speed (frames per second)	30	30	30	15
Camera Type	Analog	Digital	Digital with Strobe	High-Resolution Digital with Strobe

* Rated on a scale of 1 to 5: 1 = poor, 5 = perfect

From Table 5.1, we can see that Quick Glance 2 is available for both desktop and laptop computers. For desktop computers, a camera is mounted on the front of the monitor, so it is non-intrusive to the user. However, for laptop computers, a camera needs to be placed on the keyboard, so it may not be suitable for usability testing because it prevents the user from typing. In addition, EyeTech offers the Eye Science software which is composed of two parts: a control panel and a system developer's kit as detailed below:

    1. The Eye Science control panel features controls for:
- Adjusting the capture rate up to a maximum of 30 samples per second.
- Starting and stopping gaze capture.
- Playing back eye gaze data in real-time to illustrate the user's gaze path.
- Saving eye gaze data to a text file.
- Reading eye gaze data from a text file.

    2. The Eye Science System Developer's Kit allows a programmer to:
- Control Quick Glance through function calls from your own application.
- Use Microsoft Visual C++ and Visual Basic.
- Read gaze data directly into your software in real-time.
- Enable or disable cursor movement.
- Trigger the start and stop times of the data acquisition.
- Control the size and appearance of the Quick Glance software windows.
- Perform other miscellaneous functions.

SensoMotoric Instruments (2002) has developed various eye tracking systems which are suitable for different applications. The one most suitable for usability evaluation is the iView X system, which is available with remote interface (RED) or head mounted interface (HED). The iView X system also comes with the analysis software that provides support for:

1. Area of Interest Analysis
   - Up to 16 overlapping objects
   - Up to 256 non-overlapping objects defined by a 256 color bitmap file
2. Fixation Analysis
   - Shows the viewing path or linked fixations over a visual stimulus
   - Displays location and length of fixations over live video or still images
3. Statistical Analysis
   - Absolute and relative duration of fixations
   - Duration of fixations of any subject as percentage of a selected time interval

SR Research (2002) offers the EyeLink II system which contains a head mounted eye tracker. The EyeLink II system also includes the tracker application to be run on the host computer and the C development kit. The EyeLink Data Viewer software is optional and can be used for further data analysis.

Arrington Research (2003) has developed the ViewPoint EyeTracker system with different configurations. One of them is the remote camera system which allows a greater distance between the camera and the user's eyes. The ViewPoint EyeTracker software offers an intuitive user interface and also provides a few tools to conduct eye tracking experiments, including:

1. Stimulus Presentation
   - Present visual stimulus movies and pictures to the subject
   - Use lists to present a series of movies and/or pictures
   - Randomize stimulus presentation
2. Event Triggers
   - Trigger events when the subject looks into or out of a region of interest
   - Trigger events on a key press response
   - Timing parameters
   - Auditory cues

The ViewPoint system also comes with a software development kit and real-time/post-hoc data analysis tools.

Tobii Technology (2003) offers various eye tracking devices, including the ET-17, which is a 17-inch TFT monitor with built-in eye tracker. Also available is the ET-ClipOn, which is an eye tracker that can be attached to standard monitors, televisions, etc; it offers the same functionality as the ET-17. Regarding software, Tobii provides ClearView analysis software which includes various add-ons for different applications, including:

- VideoSync add-on: Make a digital video recording of what happens on the user's screen, and play this back as a movie with the eye-gaze data superimposed. Save your results as an .avi file. Does not require any additional hardware.
- AutomaticAOI add-on: Automatically detect objects on websites, and define areas of interest by simply clicking on the objects of interest for the study. The application will record the dynamic position of these objects, and synchronize this with eye-tracking data. A variety of statistics can be generated based on this information.
- ScriptEngine add-on: Create scripts with animated objects, slide shows etc and automatically correlate script events and positions of objects with your eye-gaze data.
- Hotspot add-on: Generate hot-spot maps to intuitively visualize eye-gaze patterns. This is done by altering the brightness of the screen contents based on the amount of

attention received. Hotspot analysis is especially powerful when used for analysis across entire groups of people.

Seeing Machines (2003a, 2003b) provides the faceLAB system which combines head, face, and eye tracking into one. The faceLAB system is non-intrusive to the user because it does not require any device to be worn by the user. Instead of the usual single camera, the faceLAB system uses dual cameras. The following quote from Seeing Machines explains how faceLAB works:

> faceLAB is a monochrome video-based tracking system, that is able to find a face in an image sequence and then home in on facial landmarks, such as the lips, nose and eyes, to obtain accurate position estimates of the features in each image. Data is then combined from two video sources (stereo), to generate 3D measurement information. Once the head-pose is located, the eye images are examined and the gaze direction is inferred from pupil orientation. (Seeing Machines, 2003a)

The faceLAB system is discussed in detail here because it was utilised in the experiment that forms part of this book. The faceLAB system was chosen because of its immediate availability and local support in Australia. The version of faceLAB used in the experiment is faceLAB 3.2.1, which contains dual cameras, PC, and accessories. The dual cameras are mounted on a stand (called Stereo-Head) as shown in Figure 5.1.

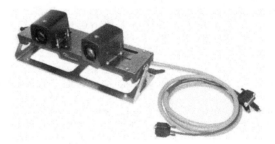

Figure 5.1   faceLAB Stereo-Head (Seeing Machines, 2003b)

The distance between the two cameras and their tilt angle can be adjusted easily according to the position of the user whose eye gaze is to be tracked. It is recommended that the distance between the cameras and the user be between 0.5 to 2.0 metres, while the tilt angle of the cameras must not exceed 15 degrees. It is best to select a user distance and a tilt angle that enable the cameras to capture the whole face of the user. Figure 5.2 depicts a recommended setup of faceLAB hardware.

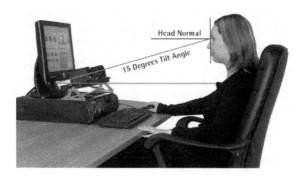

Figure 5.2 Recommended setup of faceLAB hardware (Seeing Machines, 2003b)

During the tracking process, faceLAB can measure head-pose, gaze direction, saccades, attention, what objects people are looking at, eye closure, PERCLOS fatigue measure, and eye blinks. To track the user's face and head position, faceLAB first builds a model of the user's face. This process relies on unique features of the face, such as eye and lip corners, or artificial markers that can be applied to increase tracking accuracy. Therefore, it is necessary to build a unique model for each user under specific lighting conditions and camera settings. If any of these factors change (e.g. marker position, lighting, camera tilt angle, etc.), the model previously created cannot be used any longer and a new model has to be built. It is simple to build a model as faceLAB provides a built-in semi-automated application for this purpose. The application takes snapshots of the user and allows the experimenter to select unique features of the user's face. Two types of models can be created within faceLAB: *full head* and *front-only*. While a full head model is more suitable in the case where the user's head rotates more than 30 degrees to the left or right during the tracking process, it requires more unique features to be tracked, usually around the sides of the head, e.g. ears, side-burns, earrings, etc. In addition to face/head model building, faceLAB also requires the calibration of eye gaze in order to track the user's eye gaze accurately. This can be done by having the user look into each camera for a few seconds. The following parameters can also be adjusted to increase the accuracy: pupil radius, iris radius, and eye opening. Further details of the procedures for using the faceLAB gaze tracker are provided in Chapter 7.

5.3 Web Usability Research with Eye Tracking

During the past few years, there have been a significant number of research studies concentrating on the usability of Web sites. However, only a few studies utilised the eye gaze tracking technique as a means of gathering information from users. This could be because eye tracking is a fairly new technique compared to other observation methods (e.g. videotaping, keystroke recording, etc.), and the price of most eye tracking systems available on the market is still high, starting from US$4,000. Nevertheless, it is notable that the price of eye tracking systems has decreased over time. For example, the price of one system was US$250,000 in 1988 and US$20,000 in 1996 (Joch, 1996). The functionality and usability of eye gaze analysis software is also steadily improving. Therefore, in the near future, eye tracking technologies will be more popular among usability experts in research and commercial domains as their prices become cheaper and a wider range of hardware and software products are available.

One popular approach used to analyse user's gaze behaviour is to superimpose gaze trails over a screen capture, as shown in Figure 5.3.

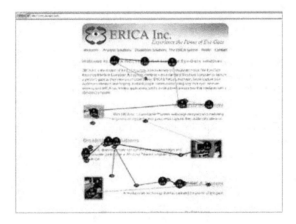

Figure 5.3   Gaze trails provided by GazeTracker (Eye Response Technologies, 2003)

For example, Newman (2001) conducted Web usability testing by using this technique. The eye tracker hardware used in Newman's study was the model 504 from Applied Science Laboratories, while the software used for the analysis was GazeTracker from Eye Response Technologies. The participants were asked to visit four Web sites: CNN; CUinfo (Cornell University); Yahoo; and Amazon, and complete different tasks on each of these sites, except for the CNN Web site where the users did not have to complete any task. The GazeTracker software automatically detected user eye movements and provided gaze trails as shown in Figure 5.4.

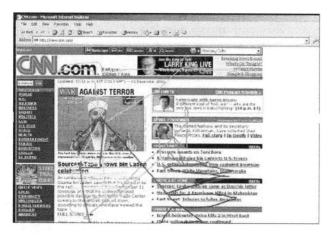

Figure 5.4   Gaze trails for CNN Web site (Newman, 2001)

The software also generated multiple graphs representing different characteristics of users' gazing behaviour. One example is a three-dimensional bar graph. The height of each LookZone represents total time spent looking at it as shown in Figure 5.5.

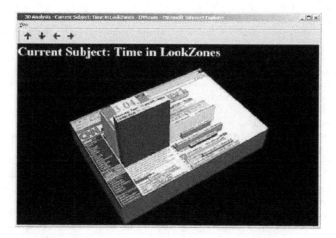

Figure 5.5   Bar graph provided by GazeTracker (Newman, 2001)

From the visual analysis of gaze trails and graphs, eye gaze patterns on the CNN Web site show that users tend to focus on new information and overlook objects that always stay the same or do not contain much information, such as the navigation bar and pictures. For the other three Web sites, it was found that the Yahoo Web site was clearly the most difficult to find information needed to complete the tasks.

In addition to Newman's (2001) study discussed above, there are also other examples of Web usability research incorporating the eye gaze tracking technique. For instance, Stanford-Poynter (2000) conducted a research project that used eye tracking to observe users while reading online news. The research was conducted using the EyeLink eye tracking system from SensoMotoric Instruments (later transferred to SR Research). The EyeLink head mounted tracking device was used in conjunction with software written by Stanford to capture both eye movements and screen content. The participants were allowed to read news on their favourite Web sites. The findings from this research included:

- At the first glance of a page, users focus on text before graphics or photos.
- Users look at banner advertisements and perceive them even though they do not click on them.
- Users scan the whole page first to find topics of their interest and then focus on them.
- Users switch back and forth between multiple Web sites instead of reading them serially.

Cowen (2001) used eye movements to evaluate the usability of the Orange company's homepages from four different countries: Belgium, India, Switzerland, and the United Kingdom. The eye tracking hardware used was SensoMotoric Instruments' Head Mounted Eyetracking Device II (HED II) with Scene Camera. The software used was iView developed by the same provider. In the experiment, participants were asked to complete two tasks on each of the four homepages. Two types of data were gathered from the experiment: performance data and eye movement data. Performance was measured by response scores and task completion times, while eye movement data was analysed using four measures: average fixation duration, number of fixations, spatial density, and total fixation duration. Then analysis of variance was performed for each measure. Inferring from the performance data analysis, the author found that there were significant interactions between the usability of a given page and the task performed on it. However, no significant interaction between page and task could be inferred from the eye movement data analysis.

Goldberg, Stimson, Lewenstein, Scott, and Wichansky (2002) conducted an eye tracking study to evaluate the usability of Oracle's Web portal prototype software. The eye tracking hardware used in this study was a SensoMotoric Instruments' EyeLink eye tracker (version 1.1), while the software used was the iView on-line analysis software. The participants were asked to complete three training tasks and six experimental tasks on custom-made Web pages, using Oracle's Web portal prototype. The screen was divided into small areas (called portlets[3]), in which Web content was displayed. The results of the study showed that for a Web page with two columns of portlets, users preferred to search horizontally across columns instead of searching vertically within a column. Another finding was that the participants did not always rely on a portlet's header bar for navigation. In addition, this study also implies several recommendations for portlet design, such as that portlets in the left column receive more attention than those in the right column and that the two most important portlets should be placed in the top two positions in the left column.

5.4 Procedures for Web Usability Evaluation with Eye Tracking

In evaluating Web usability, the eye tracking technique can be used to capture eye movements of users while they browse the Web. But first we must understand why eyes have to move at all. Because the area of maximum acuity for human eyes is quite small, we can see clearly and vividly on only a small area at a time and the rest appears blurry. So when we are faced with a large picture (such as a Web page), our eyes move around to scan small areas and get small pieces of information, then combine them to form the big picture just like solving a jigsaw puzzle.

It is also important to know which usability dimensions can be evaluated with the help of eye tracking technique. These include:

1. **Clarity/presentation:** By analysing eye movements, we are able to gain more information about user perception of the presentation on a Web page and use it for usability evaluation. For example, in Stanford-Poynter's (2000) experiment with eye tracking, it was found that users were more interested in text than graphics while they looked at Web pages. Alternative layouts can also be compared in similar fashion.

2. **Navigation support:** Different Web sites may contain different types of navigation support, and the eye tracking technique can be used to evaluate the efficiency of different navigation styles. For instance, Goldberg et al. (2002) discovered in their eye-tracking research study that users did not always rely on a portlet's header bar for navigation.

3. **Attractiveness/annoyance:** Users' eye movement data can be used to indicate the attractiveness or annoyance of specific components on a Web page, such as banner or pop-up advertisements. For example, the result of Stanford-Poynter's (2000) eye gaze tracking experiment shows that users looked at banner advertisements even though they did not click on them.

---

[3] Portlets are the visible active components end users see within their portal pages. Similar to a window in a PC desktop, each portlet owns a portion of the browser or PDA screen where it displays results. (IBM, 2003)

4. **Interaction opportunities:** Eye tracking can be used to detect whether the users realise various interaction opportunities on a Web page. For example, in the case of an image map (which is an image composed of a few clickable graphics), if the users gaze at one image map for a specific amount of time without clicking, maybe they do not realise that they can really click on it. Another example is "Mystery Meat Navigation," which is a group of unlabeled but clickable graphics (usually non-universal icons or sometimes just bullets) and the users never know where those links lead until they pass a mouse over it (Flanders, 2002). The success or failure of Mystery Meat Navigation can be tested with eye tracking in the same fashion as image maps.

The important assumption underlying the use of eye tracking as a Web usability evaluation technique is that eye movement patterns can portray the usability of a Web page. By this we assume that the users are thinking about what they are currently looking at. As a Web page is getting more usable, the pattern of eye movements should be getting simpler. This concept was emphasised by Marshall, Drapeau, and DiSciullo (2000, p. 31) as follows:

> The [...] essential measure of usability is based on the degree of confusion or hesitation that users display in trying to navigate around a website. If users find the site understandable and easy to use, they tend to navigate quickly and easily. If they have difficulty understand the logic of the site, they tend to have specific eye patterns that reveal this confusion.

However, saying whether eye movement patterns are simple or complicated is rather subjective, therefore we need to use some kind of objective (quantitative) measure. Various types of eye movement data and measures are available for usability evaluation. However, before analysis approaches are considered, it is important to understand that there are two common types of eye movements: *saccades* and *fixations*. The Applied Vision Research Unit (2004) provides definitions of saccade and fixation as follows:

> A saccade is a rapid eye movement (a jump) which is usually conjugate (i.e. both eyes move together in the same direction) and under voluntary control. Broadly speaking the purpose of these movements is to move the eyes such that images of particular areas of the visual world fall onto the fovea[4]. Saccades are therefore a major instrument of selective visual attention. [...] A fixation occurs when the eye is "stationary" between saccades and it is convenient to assume that the area imaged on to the fovea (or very near to the fovea) during a fixation is being visually attended to by the observer.

There are various types of eye movement data/measures that can be used to evaluate usability of Web site. Josephson (2002) summarised and grouped them into four categories:

1. Measures of processing
   1.1. Number of fixations

---

[4] The small area of a retina that has the greatest density of light-sensitive cells and therefore provides the highest visual acuity. Visual acuity falls off very sharply away from the fovea and so essentially we only see an object clearly and in great detail when its image falls on to the fovea.

As we can see from the list above, there are various types of measures available from the eye tracking technique. However, not all of them are suitable for every task and some of them may not be supported by most eye tracking software systems. Therefore, the following list suggests some frequently used eye movement measures with their descriptions (Josephson, 2002):

- Number of fixations: In visual search, the number of fixations is related to the number of components that the user is required to process, but not the depth of required processing. However, once the searcher has found what he/she is interested in, the number of fixations indicates the amount of interest in a visual area.

- Location of fixations: Fixations indicate one's spatial focus of attention over time. The eyes naturally fixate on areas that are surprising, salient, or important through experience.

- Fixation duration: Longer fixations imply the user is spending more time interpreting or relating the visual representation to internalized representation. Therefore, representations that require long fixations are not as meaningful to the user as those with shorter fixation durations.

- Cumulative fixation time: The total amount of fixation time on an area of interest is generally interpreted as the amount of interest a viewer has in that particular visual element. It is also interpreted as the amount of time spent processing the information.

- Scanpath length: Scanpath length is computed by summing the distance (in pixels) between gazepoint samples. Shorter scanpaths seem to indicate that the information is well-organized and information is easy to find. Lengthy scanpaths indicate less efficient scanning behavior but do not distinguish between search and information processing times.

- Scanpath duration: Scanpath duration is more related to processing complexity than to visual search efficiency, a much more relative time is spent in fixations than in saccades.

- Spatial density: Coverage of an interface due to search and processing may be captured by the spatial distribution of gazepoint samples. Evenly spread samples throughout the display indicate extensive search with an inefficient path, whereas targeted samples in a small area reflect direct and efficient search.

GazeTracker is an example of an eye tracking software system that supports several eye gaze measurements. GazeTracker was developed by Eye Response Technologies (formerly Erica, Inc.) to complement the company's ERICA hardware system. However, it may also be used in conjunction with eye tracking hardware from other providers (depending on the compatibility of the tools). The eye movement measures supported by GazeTracker are shown in Table 5.2.

Table 5.2   Eye movement measures supported by GazeTracker (Applied Science Laboratories, 2003)

Overall Metrics	LookZone Statistics
• Time span shown start (seconds) • Time span shown end (seconds) • Number of fixations • Average fixation duration (seconds) • Total time shown (seconds) • Total tracking time lost (seconds) • Total fixation duration (seconds) • Total time nonfixated excluding gaps (seconds) • Percent time lost • Percent time fixated • Percent time nonfixated • Fixation Count / Total Time • Fixation points in zones • Percent fixations in zones	• Total time in zone (seconds) • Percent time spent in zone • Fixation count • Fixation Count / Total Time in zone • Percentage of total fixations • Average fixation duration • Total fixation duration • Total time not fixated (seconds) • Percent time fixated • Percent time nonfixated • Percentage of total fixation time spent fixated • Number of fixations before first arrival • Percentage of total fixations before first arrival • Duration before first arrival • Percentage of total slide time before first arrival • Number of times zone observed

Moreover, GazeTracker is a powerful eye tracking software package because it offers three analysis options, including still image analysis, video analysis, and software analysis (with support for Web and dynamic content). For the usability evaluation of Web pages, software analysis is the most appropriate one to use. Tabbers (2002, pp. 64-65) discussed this in his thesis as follows:

> In Application Analysis, the program combines the input from eye-tracking systems like ERICA, ASL or SMI with information about the activities of the user of a computer application, like keystrokes and mouse clicks. In this way, all activities on the screen can be related to gaze position data, which gives the opportunity to track eye movements in several applications simultaneously and even control for scrolling behaviour in web browsers. Moreover, specific areas of interest, called LookZones, can be defined for separate windows and for web pages. These LookZones provide metrics concerning how long and how often a test subject observed different areas of interest. After recording, the data including the interactions of the user with the applications can be replayed, and can be displayed as a gaze trail, which depicts the scan path of a test subject, superimposed on an application window. The program also provides other

graphical analysis methods, such as bar charts in Excel based on the LookZone data or three-dimensional views of the application window with the time duration of the eye-tracking data in different regions depicted in the z-dimension. GazeTracker also allows experimenters to export the data to text files or to Microsoft Excel for further statistical analysis in other statistical software packages.

As discussed previously in this chapter, GazeTracker is not the only tool available on the market. Several other eye tracking systems are readily available to choose from. Different systems offer different features and pricing, hence usability evaluators are responsible for the selection of tools suitable for their usability evaluations. Once an appropriate eye gaze tracking tool is chosen and acquired, the installation and calibration of eye tracking hardware and software are usually required. Then, Web usability evaluation procedures begin with asking the participant to visit Web sites to be evaluated and having the participant look around the sites as they would normally and/or complete some predefined tasks. The eye tracking system automatically detects eye movements of the participant while browsing the Web sites and then provides information regarding several eye gaze measurements for further statistical analyses. Complementary data such as gaze trails and graphs may also be presented to the usability evaluator, so the evaluator can use visual inspection to analyse these gaze trails and graphs. Usually, gaze trails and graphs of multiple Web pages are compared to estimate their relative usability. In addition, quantitative analysis of gaze trails can also be made, but the evaluator might have to choose a suitable algorithm and develop a program specifically for it, because this type of analysis is usually not included in the eye tracking software package commercially available on the market.

5.5   Validation of Eye Gaze Point Estimates

In addition to several quantitative eye gaze measures previously discussed, eye gaze points representing small areas on the screen where the user is looking at during the period of eye gaze tracking experiment could also be analysed. Different eye tracking systems provide different methods and levels of support for eye gaze point estimates. For instance, GazeTracker provides the observer with *GazeTrail*, a diagram showing connected gaze points over a period of time superimposed over a stimulus, and *LookZone*, an area of interest (customisable by the observer) whose duration and order in which the user is looking at could be obtained (Eye Response Technologies, 2003). However, the accuracy of eye gaze point estimates is rarely validated. Several eye tracking systems leave it up to the observer to determine the accuracy, often by comparing the estimates to the points believed to be looked at by the user. This method is rather subjective and tedious, especially when a large number of participants are involved in the experiment and/or each experimental period lasts longer than a few minutes. Therefore, the validation of eye gaze point estimates could instead be integrated into the eye tracking system. This could be done by displaying stimuli on different parts of the screen (one by one) and having the user look at them serially, so that the system could determine distances between the stimuli and the estimated gaze points (called "displacement vectors"), and adapt itself accordingly to provide higher accuracy. The stimuli presented should be meaningful to the user, so that it is certain that the user would look at them. For example, numbers, letters, or figures could be used, and the user should be required to read them aloud, to show that they are really looking at these stimuli.

Displacement vectors are the indicator of the accuracy of eye gaze point estimates. Each vector has a direction that points from the estimated gaze point to the actual gaze point, and can be represented by a length/angle pair (e.g. 2cm, 120°) or an x-y coordinate (e.g. -1x+1.732y), as shown in Figure 5.6.

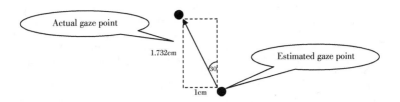

Figure 5.6   Example of displacement vector

There are two major factors contributing to the inaccuracy of gaze point estimates and hence the magnitude of the displacement vector: *space* and *time*. By *space*, it is meant that at a specific point in time, displacement vectors may or may not be the same for all positions (pixels) on the screen. And by *time*, it is meant that the displacement vector of a specific point on the screen may also change over time. Therefore, in order to design a self-adaptive eye tracking system, these two factors should be taken into account for accuracy correction purposes. For example, at the beginning of the tracking, it may not be known whether the displacement vectors of different points on the screen will differ by how much or whether they will change over time. Thus, at first, a number of stimuli should be presented on as many parts of the screen as possible, and the presentation should be repeated periodically and often (e.g. every five minutes). When the tracking progresses, if the displacement vectors of different points on the screen do not differ by much, the number of stimuli in each presentation could be reduced. And if the displacement vector of a specific point on the screen does not change too often over time, the interval between each stimuli presentation could be made longer, therefore involving less interruption to the user.

If the eye tracking system automatically adjusts itself using periodical presentations of stimuli on the screen as previously discussed, it is expected that the effects of the influential factors on estimated eye gaze point accuracy could be kept at a minimum at all times during the period of experiment. However, at present, only a few (if any) eye tracking systems have the ability to do this, as most eye tracking systems available on the market allow calibration only at the beginning of the experiment. Furthermore, the calibration is usually done without verification for the accuracy. For example, the faceLAB eye tracking system displays stimuli (white dots) on the screen and captures user's eye positions when the user looks at different parts of the screen and uses this information to estimate the user's gaze points. However, once the calibration has finished, the accuracy is not verified in anyway, as the only option available is to recalibrate once again if the estimated gaze spot does not correspond well to the actual gaze spot of the user (as judged by the observer). At any rate, it is promising that the next generation of eye tracking systems will be able to incorporate the ability to self-adjust their estimated gaze point accuracy within the near future.

5.6 Conclusion

This chapter has discussed the role of eye tracking in usability evaluation, specifically for the Web. Various eye tracking tools have been presented as well as examples of related Web usability evaluation projects. This chapter concluded with the discussion of procedures commonly undertaken to evaluate Web sites using the eye tracking technique. Although eye gaze tracking is gaining more popularity among usability experts, other usability evaluation techniques should not be totally disregarded. Instead, they could be used as a complement to the eye tracking technique, as appropriate.

6

Macromedia Flash and the Web

6.1 Introduction

Since the development of the Web in the early 1990s, many Web publishing platforms have been made available, including HyperText Markup Language (HTML) and its successor Extensible HyperText Markup Language (XHTML), Dynamic HyperText Markup Language (DHTML), Macromedia Flash, Macromedia Shockwave, Java, and many more. However, only two of them have become standards accepted by most Web users and developers alike; they are HTML and Macromedia Flash. When HTML is mentioned here, it covers all of its variants, including XHTML (a stricter version of HTML that can run on various platforms, e.g. mobile phones and PDAs) and other Web development technologies which also generate HTML-like Web pages, e.g. ASP (Active Server Pages) and PHP (Hypertext Preprocessor). HTML has long been known as the standard format for publishing of content on the Web because it was introduced at the same time as the Web itself. However, standard HTML has limited capabilities for managing interactive or animated content, so a few other technologies have emerged as extensions to standard HTML. Macromedia Flash is one of these add-ons, and the most successful, because it does not have cross-browser and cross-platform compatibility problem like DHTML, and it is more stable than Java applets (McGregor, 2003). Because of its ever-increasing functionality and popularity, the role of Flash has gradually shifted from being an add-on to becoming a replacement of HTML, as can be seen from the increasing number of Web sites created entirely in Flash.

At present, all available PC Web browsers (e.g. Microsoft Internet Explorer, Netscape Navigator, Opera, etc.) support HTML, therefore all Web users can view Web sites developed in HTML immediately. On the other hand, not all Web browsers are Flash-enabled; some browsers need to download Flash player plug-in software before they can display Flash Web sites properly. However, the percentage of Web users equipped with a Flash-enabled browser is reasonably high. According to NPD Online's recent survey (conducted in March 2003), they constitute 79.3% to 98.9% of all Web users, depending on their geographic location and Flash version supported (Macromedia, 2003a). Even though these statistics show that Flash Web sites can be viewed by most online users, they do not provide any ground for us to believe that Flash technology is indeed welcomed by these users. However, there is evidence suggesting that Flash has been warmly embraced by many Web developers. In the year 2002, it was reported that 25% of all Web sites used Flash content (Network World Fusion, 2002).

6.2   History of the Web, HTML, and Flash

The Web and HTML began at the same time. The story began when Tim Berners-Lee who worked at CERN (Conseil Européen pour la Recherche Nucléaire) had an idea of creating a distributed information system where everyone could gain access to a large amount of information stored separately at several places around the world, without the need to know its real physical locations. Some of the most significant features of this system are that multiple pieces of information within the system can be linked together using hypertext and that users of the system can easily add their own information to the system. Berners-Lee submitted the proposal containing his idea to CERN in 1989 and after a few revisions (with help from Robert Cailliau who also worked at CERN), the World Wide Web was born.

HTML was invented by Berners-Lee as the standard publishing format of information on the Web. HTML was largely based on SGML (Standard Generalised Markup Language), which at that time was already an ISO standard markup language. From then until now, there have been various versions of HTML as well as the introduction of XHTML (the most widely used XHTML version at the time of writing is version 1.0), and later versions are always supersets of previous versions (i.e. provide backward compatibility). During 1990-1995, HTML was the only standard format for Web publishing, therefore it was utilised in all Web sites. Even though HTML offers the powerful ability to publish text and still images on the Web, it provides limited support for animations (through animated GIFs) and sounds (through embedded sound files). Therefore, a few add-ons to HTML have emerged to provide developers with higher capability to publish interactive animations on the Web, one of which was FutureSplash Animator which later became known as Flash.

Jonathan Gay (2003) was the owner of a company named FutureWave. Working for his own company, Gay created a software application called FutureSpash Animator, which was made commercially available in 1996. It is a tool used to create two-dimensional graphic animation that can be sent over the Internet and displayed on the Netscape Web browser. Major clients of FutureSpash Animator included Microsoft and Disney, thus providing FutureSpash with success and fame. Macromedia, the creator of Shockwave (a different technology which can also be used for Web animation), heard about FutureSpash and saw its potential to be the most feasible technology for Web animation (as Shockwave files were much larger). Therefore, in the same year that FutureSpash Animator was released, Macromedia decided to take over Gay's company FutureWave, along with its most talked about product, FutureSplash Animator. After the takeover, FutureSpash Animator was renamed Macromedia Flash 1.0 and Gay has been working with Macromedia ever since. Until now, Macromedia has been developing Flash continuously, releasing seven major versions. At the time of writing, the latest version is Flash MX 2004 (version 7), which was released in 2003.

One of the major characteristics of Flash technology is that it utilises vector graphics, in contrast to the raster graphics used in animated GIFs. Vector graphics (object-oriented graphics) store data as mathematical formulae and use them to draw objects on the screen when activated. The major benefit of vector graphics is that they consume only a small amount of disk space because data kept in vector files consists mostly of mathematical formulae (which are text). Furthermore, vector graphics can be displayed on the screen at any size without losing quality, so they will look exactly the same on every computer at any screen resolution. On the other hand, a raster (also called bitmap) image file (e.g. GIF, JPG, BMP, etc.) stores data for each of the image's pixels. Therefore, the larger the image is, the bigger its bitmap file has to be. Besides, a bitmap image does not look the same on every computer; it looks bigger on a computer with a smaller screen resolution. Although vector imaging has advantages over raster imaging with respect to file size and viewing consistency (i.e. independent screen resolution), it also has major drawbacks: vector imaging can only be used for Bezier or B-spline curves, which are lines defined by mathematical formulae (examples include geometric shapes and TrueType or PostScript fonts); and it cannot be used for real-life representations such as those taken with a camera. Therefore, Macromedia Flash supports both vector and raster images, which means that not all Flash Web sites are small and fast-loading, hence the efficiency of the Web site depends on the proportion of vector/raster images used in the site.

6.3   The Uses of Flash on the Web

Since its first version release, Macromedia Flash has been employed by a significant number of Web sites around the world. Many commercial and personal Web sites use it in one way or another. There appear to be three main purposes of incorporating Flash elements into a Web site:

1. **Flash for animation/presentation:** This used to be the primary usage of Flash a few years ago. Many Web sites used Flash for displaying an animation sequence (TV-like) or a presentation (PowerPoint-like). Users are provided with no control of Flash elements except for play buttons, such as forward or back. This type of Flash animation has been used extensively as a way of introducing users to a Web site (commonly called "Flash Intro"). Contents of Flash Intro usually include: company or Web site name; logo; motto; products/services offered; and anything else that helps create the brand image. These components are arranged in an

animation sequence with optional sound effects and/or voice narration. Most Flash Intros can be skipped by the users, if they want to, by clicking the "Skip Intro" link (if provided)—primarily intended for repeat users of the Web site. Over the past few years, Flash Intro has been used so prevalently that the expression "Skip Intro" is sometimes considered synonymous with Flash technology. However, the use of Flash Intro has declined recently due to the fact that it provides little additional value to the Web site and users do not like it because they have to click "Skip Intro" every time they revisit the Web site or else they have to go through the whole animation routine again. Apart from Flash Intro, Flash technology is often used for the presentation of slide shows on the Web in the same fashion as PowerPoint is used, but Flash allows more integration with the Web than PowerPoint does.

2. **Flash for navigation:** Flash elements can be used to support Web site navigation as well. Most of the time, a Flash Intro is expanded to include navigation aids at the end, i.e. after the users have been presented with the animation sequence (or more often, after they click "Skip Intro"), they are provided with links to various sections on the Web site. Flash technology enables links to be responsive to user's mouse movements/clicks in the same fashion as JavaScript and Java Applets. These features usually include: rollover buttons; drop-down/expandable menus; and sound effects.

3. **Flash for all content:** At present, there are an increasing number of Web sites created entirely in Flash. This purpose is different from the two discussed above because Flash technology is not used as a complement to HTML, but rather as a replacement for HTML. This type of Web site is the main concern of this research project because of its increasing popularity and various usability issues that come with it.

6.4 Flash and Usability

In the year 2000, usability guru Jakob Nielsen published in his Alertbox[1] column an article regarding Macromedia Flash technology, as used primarily in various Web sites at that time. His article was entitled, alarmingly, "Flash: 99% Bad," and he explained the reason for this harsh judgement, as follows:

> About 99% of the time, the presence of Flash on a website constitutes a usability disease. Although there are rare occurrences of good Flash design (it even adds value on occasion), the use of Flash typically lowers usability. In most cases, we would be better off if these multimedia objects were removed. Flash tends to degrade websites for three reasons: it encourages design abuse, it breaks with the Web's fundamental interaction principles, and it distracts attention from the site's core value. (Nielsen, 2000)

---

[1] Online bi-weekly Web-based column focusing on usability issues written by Jakob Nielsen

In his article, Nielsen pointed out various usability issues that arose because of the introduction of Flash technology. He mentioned the following major problems inherent in Flash-enabled Web sites at that time: unnecessary intro/animation; lack of user control (more TV-like experience); and nonstandard scrollbar. He also noted that it was not that the Flash technology itself was inherently bad, but rather that Web designers already had an inclination to break usability rules and Flash just enabled them to do so more easily. For example, it is easy to create nonstandard scrollbars in Flash but it is impossible to do so using plain HTML.

In the year 2002, after Macromedia had received considerable negative feedback concerning Flash (the most prominent being Nielsen's article discussed above), they decided to seek help from a usability expert, who turned out to be the same Jakob Nielsen who wrote the article "Flash: 99% Bad" two years before. Therefore, in June 2002, a few months after the release of Flash MX (Flash version 6), Macromedia and the Nielsen Norman Group (a company founded by Jakob Nielsen and Donald Norman) formed a strategic partnership focusing on the improvement of Flash usability (Macromedia, 2002). Their ultimate goal was to make Flash Web sites "100% good" instead of "99% bad." As part of that agreement, Nielsen developed a number of usability guidelines for Web design/development with Flash MX[2]. In addition, Nielsen contributed to one of the major changes in Flash MX from the previous version; Flash MX was shipped with a standard set of interface components (e.g. scrollbars, buttons, etc.) so that Flash designers could use them to increase consistency across Web sites.

Since the year 2002, Macromedia has encouraged Web designers/developers around the world to use Flash MX to create Web sites entirely in Flash. However, the benefit of switching the Web from HTML-based to Flash-based is still obscure. Although Flash technology enables more application-like Web sites and higher integration of animated contents, the usability of Web sites created entirely in Flash has not yet been determined. Becker (2002) wrote about this "Flash everywhere" situation as follows:

> One promised pay-off is easier-to-use transaction sites with content that, through Flash-enabled browsers, can be updated selectively rather than having to redraw the entire page every time new data is submitted. Another pay-off is video clips that don't require a separate browser window. But critics say a Flash-everywhere approach carries hidden potential liabilities that could stifle innovation. [...] Flash can also limit the sharing of Web information. Flash pages can't be easily indexed, making them inaccessible to search engines. And because everything happens within the same browser window, there's no way to link to specific parts of a Flash site.

From the year 2003, it is evident that the "Flash everywhere" phenomenon is becoming more popular with Web site developers. Many Web sites have been created entirely in Flash, while others use a combination of Flash and HTML. McGregor (2003) has provided guidelines regarding when to use Flash or HTML as follows:

---

[2] Commercially available at http://www.nngroup.com/reports/flash/

- When to use Macromedia Flash; if these elements are important to the project, use Macromedia Flash: animation, sound, rich interactivity, compatibility across browsers, stability across platforms, server independent publishing (CDs, kiosks).
- When to use HTML; if these elements are important to the project, use HTML: long sections of text data, frequent updates (both design and content), legibility, largest possible audience, dynamic formatting of text, accessibility.

However, it is commonly found that many Web designers/developers do not utilise a combination of Flash and HTML as per the criteria above, but instead, they use only one or the other for the entire Web site. This might be because they consider that it would take longer to develop a Web site by interweaving the two approaches.

It is also useful to consider the suitability of Flash usage as contingent upon Web site purpose. For example, the categories of Web site purpose suggested by Turk (2001) are:

1. Communication (e-mail; discussion lists; chat groups)
2. Information (e.g. educational material; news)
3. Entertainment (e.g. games; gambling; pornography)
4. Services (e.g. search engines; software libraries; counseling)
5. Electronic commerce / marketing (business-customer and business-business)

It can be clearly seen that, according to their intended purpose, Web sites in some categories above may be more suitable for Flash than Web sites in other categories. For instance, communication and services Web sites are rarely found implemented in Flash because of their needs for frequent updates and large text display. On the other hand, most entertainment Web sites utilise Flash because it provides easy integration of animation and sound, which are the main features for entertainment purposes. Information and e-commerce/marketing Web sites are somewhere in between, depending on the individual Web site's purpose and target audience. Because Web site purpose can influence the usability of Flash Web sites, it is also considered in this book and discussed in the following section.

6.5 Usability Research Issues Regarding Flash Technology

Within the past few years, there have been various changes in Web site design and development. Discussed earlier in this chapter, one major change is the introduction of Flash technology as an alternative platform for the delivery of Web content. According to Macromedia, the marketer of Flash technology, Flash enables the delivery of "highly visual interactive content" through the Web (Macromedia, 2003b). Although the benefits of Flash have not yet been clearly investigated, many developers have rushed to offer the Flash version of their Web sites to the public, mostly due to the freshness of Flash technology and the impression that Flash can somehow make their Web sites "alive," and therefore attract more visitors. But since Flash requires more bandwidth and higher user hardware specifications, some users may experience difficulties viewing Flash-enabled Web sites. Therefore, at present many Web sites offer both Flash and HTML versions of their Web sites to the users.

This phenomenon can be seen by the fact that a search for the phrase "Flash version" on Google[3] search engine returned more than 300,000 results (in July 2004). Some examples of well-known Web sites which offer both Flash and HTML versions to the users can be found in Appendix 6A.

This is the trend for now, but the future is still unclear. The current situation where two platforms (Flash and HTML) are offered concurrently may soon have to be eliminated because of the double maintenance cost involved. So, will Flash eventually replace HTML Web pages? The key issue underlying this question is usability. Users of Web sites should be the ones who determine which one has to go: Flash or HTML, and usability is the key determinant. However, there have been very few comparative studies of Flash and HTML Web sites focusing on usability, in spite of the increasing controversy regarding this issue.

Therefore, this research study addresses the issue by conducting usability evaluations of Flash and HTML versions of the same set of Web sites. It is critical that such research employs a methodology which clearly addresses the research issues; it must be able to demonstrate key usability differences between alternative versions of Web sites. Based on the research reported in Chapters 2 to 5, it was decided to use two different usability evaluation techniques: (1) contingent heuristic approach (WUCET questionnaire) and (2) eye gaze tracking (faceLAB). Other independent variables that might affect the usability score, particularly (1) user's gender; (2) user's previous experience with computers and the Web; and (3) user's Internet connection speed, were also considered. Hypothesised trends will be discussed and formal hypotheses will then be listed.

Users' gender and computer/Web experience have been selected as independent variables for this research because it is hypothesised that they are the key factors that may significantly influence the way a user perceives the usability of Web sites, especially when Flash technology is used. It is hypothesised that male users prefer flashy animated graphics and sounds, which are more pervasive in Flash Web sites than in HTML Web sites. It is further hypothesised that users with more computer/Web experience may feel frustrated with animated graphics and sounds in Flash Web sites because these components may distract them from getting their work done, and their experience dulls the impact of flashy graphics. On the other hand, users with less computer/Web experience may find that Flash provides more audio-visual presentations (than HTML) and therefore helps them use Web sites more easily.

Another factor that might contribute to the perceived usability of a Web site is the speed of Internet connection. As Flash Web sites are more multimedia-oriented than HTML-only Web sites, they tend to include more graphics, sounds, and animations. This usually makes Flash Web sites slower to load than HTML counterparts, which could be easily noticeable by users with slow Internet connection (dial-up). On the other hand, several sections of Flash Web sites are usually downloaded together, compared to HTML Web sites where only one page can be downloaded at a time. Therefore, users may feel that, although Flash Web sites seem to load more slowly at first, after the site is fully loaded, it can be

---

[3] http://www.google.com

browsed faster than HTML Web sites. Before the experiment, it was unknown which of the two effects had stronger impact on usability, so it was hypothesised neutrally that users with a slower Internet connection might see greater difference in usability between the Flash and HTML versions of a Web site than users with a faster Internet connection.

In addition to user characteristics and Internet connection speed, Web site purpose also plays an important role in usability evaluation. Different types of Web sites have different types of content (text and graphics), different graphical styles, different use scenarios and user objectives. Thus different aspects of usability are of greater significance and it is speculated that there might be some significant relationship between the type of Web site, its usability (as perceived by the users), and whether Flash or HTML was used. According to Turk (2000, 2001), there are five categories of Web sites that could be considered in this context: communication, information, entertainment, services, and e-commerce/marketing. However, this study utilised only three of them: (1) information; (2) entertainment; and (3) e-commerce, because Flash technology is more likely to be found on Web sites in these three categories than in the other two.

The following research questions and their corresponding hypotheses are addressed in this study:

Q1: Is there is a difference in usability of the Flash and HTML versions of a Web site?

H1: The Flash version of a Web site provides higher usability than the HTML version.

Q2: Does users' gender affect their perception of the comparative usability of the Flash vs. HTML versions of a Web site?

H2: Male users prefer the Flash version of a Web site (over the HTML version) to a greater extent than do female users.

Q3: Does users' computer/Web experience affect their perception of the comparative usability of the Flash vs. HTML versions of a Web site?

H3: Users with shorter computer/Web experience prefer the Flash version of a Web site (over the HTML version) to a greater extent than do users with longer computer/Web experience.

Q4: Does users' Internet connection speed affect their perception of the comparative usability of the Flash vs. HTML versions of a Web site?

H4: Users with slower Internet connection speed see the difference in usability between the Flash and HTML versions of a Web site to a greater extent than do users with faster Internet connection speed.

Q5: Does the category of a Web site (information, entertainment, e-commerce) affect the comparative usability of the Flash vs. HTML versions of the Web site?

H5: The category of a Web site (information, entertainment, e-commerce) affects the comparative usability of the Flash vs. HTML versions of the Web site.

Q6: Does the version of a Web site visited (Flash or HTML) affect users' inclination and ability to perform tasks (use scenarios) within Web site, as reflected by the task completion score?

H6:   The version of a Web site visited (Flash or HTML) affects users'
      inclination and ability to perform tasks (use scenarios) within Web
      site, as reflected by the task completion score.

6.6   Conclusion

This chapter has discussed the role of Flash on the Web. It has been found that many Web sites utilise Flash technology; some Web sites use Flash as an add-on, while some Web sites are created entirely in Flash. However, true usability of Flash Web sites is still in doubt. Therefore, usability evaluations of Web sites developed entirely in Flash should be undertaken as compared to HTML-only Web sites, and the comparative study of these two approaches forms part of this research. Two usability evaluation methods discussed earlier (contingent heuristic approach and eye gaze tracking) are used to compare Flash and HTML Web sites. Detailed information about the research design and methodology will be discussed in the following chapter.

7

Research Design and Methodology

7.1 Introduction

In the previous chapter, six hypotheses were proposed regarding the usability issues of Flash vs. HTML Web sites. In order to test these hypotheses, usability comparisons between Flash and HTML Web sites have been made by utilising both the contingent heuristic approach and the eye gaze tracking technique, as discussed in Chapters 4 and 5, respectively.

This research study utilised a pilot study and two major experiments: Phase One experiment—usability survey (to implement a contingent heuristic approach) and Phase Two experiment—eye gaze tracking. The time schedule for this research study is summarised in Table 7.1.

Table 7.1   Research time schedule

Month	Activities
1	• Prepared research plan
2	• Reviewed WUCET application
3-4	• Prepared protocol for pilot study of usability survey • Set up online usability survey
5	• Conducted pilot study of usability survey
6-7	• Revised usability survey • Prepared protocol for Phase One experiment (usability survey)
8	• Conducted Phase One experiment • Prepared protocol for Phase Two experiment (eye gaze tracking)
9	• Preliminary data analysis of Phase One experiment • Set up laboratory for Phase Two experiment
10	• Conducted Phase Two experiment
11	• Detailed data analysis of Phase One experiment
12-13	• Data analysis of Phase Two experiment
14	• Interpreted and summarised research findings

The detailed research design and methodology for each phase are discussed in the following sections.

7.2   Quantitative and Qualitative Data

Research is a systematic process of acquiring new knowledge, which is based upon some form of empirical evidence (Shanks, Rouse, and Arnott, 1993). However, before the research process is discussed further, the philosophy behind all research must be discussed first. It has long been known and widely accepted that there are two main types of research, categorised by its underlying philosophy: *positivist* and *interpretivist*. Positivist research approaches are objective and empirical, while interpretivist research approaches are more subjective, based on interpretation of a range of evidence or data. Nonetheless, these two camps are not mutually exclusive. The research approach that anyone would take depends on their philosophical assumptions, ranging from experiment (the most positivist) to conceptual study (the most interpretivist). Research studies based on pure positivism or interpretivism are rarely found. On the other hand, most research studies utilise both positivist and interpretivist methods to different extents. For the research in this book, experiments and surveys were utilised. Although these two techniques are considered more positivist than interpretivist, because they depend highly on statistical analyses of quantitative data, interpretivism can also add value to the research if qualitative data is used appropriately to explain some phenomena that could not be answered adequately with quantitative data alone. Therefore, recorded comments from participants in the research can be used to indicate useful paths for future research and to illustrate results obtained from quantitative analysis.

Survey research is a way of doing research by collecting data from a representative sample (a subset of the population) and statistically analysing that data in order to derive answers to research questions. The validity of survey research depends largely on how the sample is chosen. The researcher has to select the sample carefully so that it can represent the whole population. The size of the sample has to be taken into account as well. If the sample size is too small, it may not be able to represent the actual population, but if it is too large, the survey may not be feasible because the data is difficult to collect. Most surveys are quantitative and try to answer descriptive questions or look at causal relationships, but sometimes qualitative surveys are also useful because they can provide explanations for various issues that otherwise cannot be answered quantitatively. Surveys can be conducted by mail, personal interview, telephone, and more recently, on the Internet, depending on their suitability for the research.

After research data has been collected from various sources (e.g. surveys, experiments, etc.), it has to be analysed carefully and presented in a suitable form, otherwise, the results will be useless to the readers, and worse yet, the researchers may be unable to answer their intended research questions at all. Therefore, data analysis is a very important phase of the research. There are two techniques that can be used to analyse research data: quantitative and qualitative. Quantitative techniques involve the numerical representation and manipulation of data in order to describe and explain the phenomenon reflected by this data, whereas qualitative techniques involve the non-numerical examination and interpretation of data in order to discover the subjacent explanations and patterns of interrelationship. Quantitative and qualitative techniques are generally associated with deductive and inductive approaches, respectively. The deductive approach starts with an assumption (hypothesis) and then supports it by analysing empirical evidence, while the inductive approach starts with observations that lead to a new assumption. When a quantitative analysis is applied, numerical estimates and statistical inferences obtained from a representative sample of the real population are often used. On the other hand, in qualitative analysis narrative descriptions and continuous comparisons are usually exploited in order to understand the populations or situations that are being studied.

The differences between quantitative analysis carried out under standardised conditions and qualitative analysis aiming at understanding a phenomenon in a natural context have caused a barrier between researchers following different analytical disciplines for a long time. This may be disadvantageous especially for research that relates to long-standing problems. Rather than neglecting or defending one paradigm in particular, it is possible and more advantageous to combine both quantitative and qualitative techniques and use them in a less conventional way. In other words, it is possible to describe the observable facts in the real world in a quantitative way and at the same time collect qualitative evidence within a predefined experimental context. Therefore, in the research study that forms part of this book, a combination of these two analysis techniques was utilised to emphasise that quantitative and qualitative techniques can and should coexist as complementary tools of research. The two approaches are reflected in different stages of the research process to provide a synergistic combination of data relevant to the research hypotheses.

7.3 Pilot Study of Usability Survey

The purpose of this pilot study was to determine if the usability survey prepared for Phase One of the experiment was suitable. The pilot study was conducted with five participants, three of whom were undergraduate students in the School of Information Technology, Murdoch University. The other two participants were professional Web/graphic designers. Detailed procedures (Appendix 7A) were given to each participant and they were allowed one month to complete the survey. However, the survey could not be stopped and resumed, so it was required to be finished in one session. The survey was implemented as a Web-based survey using the adaptation of an open-source tool, PHPSurveyor [1] version 0.98rc3. The advantage of this tool is that it utilises PHP scripts and a MySQL database, which are reasonably fast, reliable, and supported by most Web servers. In addition, this tool allowed the creation of a private survey, which was suitable for this study. A private survey differs from a public survey in that it requires the contributors to the survey to have tokens in order to access the survey. Each participant was e-mailed a link that included a unique token to be used for the survey. In addition, each link (token) could only be used once, i.e. when the survey was completed, the link was automatically disabled.

When a link in the e-mail they received was clicked, the participants were directed to the first part of the survey, which contained some background demographic questions. The following questions were asked:

- Age (years)
- Gender
- Computer experience (years)
- Web experience (years)
- Computer usage (hours per week)
- Web usage (hours per week)

The last two questions (computer and Web usage) were included as objective measures of experience, as the number of years alone could not represent users' experience adequately. After these background questions were completed, each participant visited two Web sites in each category (information, entertainment, and e-commerce), i.e. a total of six Web sites, and completed predefined tasks (use scenarios) for each Web site. The following is the list of Web sites used in the study:

1. Information Web sites:
   - Full Sail[2] (site A)
   - Australians At War[3] (site B)
2. Entertainment Web sites:
   - Escaflowne[4] (site C)

---

[1] http://phpsurveyor.sourceforge.net

[2] http://www.fullsail.com

[3] http://www.australiansatwar.gov.au/throughmyeyes/select.asp

- Disturbed[5] (site D)
3. E-commerce Web sites:
- Chronicle Books[6] (site E)
- Perceptron[7] (site F)

While browsing the Web sites, the participants were presented with an on-screen timer so that they could note elapsed time from the beginning to the end of the tasks. This timer was implemented using JavaScript because it is supported by most Web browsers. After the participants finished all tasks for each Web site, they were required to complete a Web usability questionnaire for that Web site, and then continue to the next Web site. The Web usability questionnaires used in the survey were obtained from the WUCET (Website Usability Contingent Evaluation Tool) developed by Dunstan (2003), as discussed in Chapter 4. Since WUCET is a contingency-based tool, the questions were different for each Web site, depending on the Web site purpose and user characteristics (for the intended site audience), as shown in Table 7.2.

Table 7.2   Web sites used in the experiment categorised by intended user characteristics and primary site purpose

Web Site	Intended User Characteristics					Primary Web Site Purpose
	Age	Culture	Disabilities	Education	Web/IT Experience	
A. Full Sail	Young	Western	None	Secondary	General	Information
B. Australians At War	General	Western	None	General	General	
C. Escaflowne	Young	Asian	None	General	General	Entertainment
D. Disturbed	General	Western	None	General	General	
E. Chronicle Books	General	General	None	General	General	E-Commerce
F. Perceptron	Middle-Aged	General	None	Tertiary/Post	General	

The usability questions which were obtained from WUCET and used for each Web site can be found in Appendix 7B. In addition to WUCET questions, the participants also had to submit the time they used to complete the tasks for each Web site and also had an option to provide any further comments about the usability of each Web site. The survey was completed when each participant had completed all tasks and questionnaires for all six Web sites.

Each Web site in the experiment has both Flash and HTML versions. In the pilot study, three participants were randomly assigned to view Flash version of the

---

[4] http://www.escamovie.com

[5] http://www.disturbed1.com

[6] http://www.chroniclebooks.com

[7] http://www.perceptron.com

Web sites, while the other two were assigned to view HTML version. After the survey had been completed, participants submitted their thoughts regarding the utility and usability of the survey to the researcher. Feedback from the participants was considered and some changes were made to the survey to make it more effective and efficient. The revised version of the survey was used in the Phase One experiment and will be discussed in the next section.

7.4 Experimental Design for the Phase One Experiment (Usability Survey)

The Phase One experiment was conducted three months after the pilot study. It has many aspects similar to the pilot study, but there are also some changes, as detailed below:

1. From the pilot study, it was found that loading speed of Web sites has an impact on survey responses. Therefore, the following question was added to the first part of the survey (background information):

   What is the speed of your Internet connection?
   - 56K or slower (e.g. dial-up)
   - 64K - 128K (e.g. ISDN)
   - 256K or faster (e.g. DSL, cable, T1)
   - Don't know

2. Some of the participants in the pilot study stated that they accidentally switched from the Flash to HTML version of a Web site, or vice versa, during the survey because they were not aware of the implications of doing so. In the Phase One experiment, the participants were explicitly told that they were about to view Flash or HTML Web sites and therefore must not switch version under any circumstance.

3. Some participants in the pilot study reported that they did not complete some tasks for some Web sites, but this information was not reflected in the responses. Therefore, in the Phase One experiment, the participants also had to answer five questions for each Web site, so the task completion rate could be measured.

4. Escaflowne Web site (site C) was replaced by Hikki Web site[8] because the former site was not accessible (server down) when the Phase One experiment took place. Disturbed Web site (site D) was replaced by Madonna Web site[9] because after the pilot study was conducted, this Web site was totally redesigned by the owner so that it was not suitable for the Phase One experiment. Screen capture of the front page of all six Web sites (both Flash and HTML versions) utilised in the experiment can be found in Appendix 7C.

---

[8] http://www.toshiba-emi.co.jp/hikki/

[9] http://www.madonna.com

5. The online survey tool (PHPSurveyor) was upgraded from version 0.98rc3 to version 0.98rc8, thus improving security and performance.

For the Phase One experiment, 43 participants were recruited. All of the participants were Murdoch University undergraduate students studying a unit about Human-Computer Interaction, including Web site usability evaluation techniques. All participants had previous experience using computers and the Web. Similar to the pilot study, the Phase One survey was made available online (Web-based) so the experimental protocol was self-administered by the participants on their own computers with Internet access. Each participant was given detailed procedures (Appendix 7D) to complete the experiment by themselves in their own time. However, the researcher could be contacted by e-mail at any time to provide assistance to the participants, if needed.

Of the 43 participants, 20 were assigned to view the Flash version of the Web sites, while the remaining 23 were assigned to view the HTML version. Therefore, there were two groups of participants:

- Group A: Participants who visited the Flash version of the Web sites
- Group B: Participants who visited the HTML version of the Web sites

The participants were randomly assigned to either group by the researcher, and then they were informed by e-mail and given the survey link according to their group.

7.5 Method of Data Analysis for the Phase One Experiment

The main independent variable in this study is Web implementation technology, which is measured using a nominal scale and, for the purpose of this study, has two possible values: Flash or HTML, i.e. mixed (hybrid) implementation cases are not considered. The dependent variables are usability scores from WUCET questionnaires, which are measured on a five-point Likert scale. Other independent variables that may affect the usability scores of Web sites are also included as follows:

- User's characteristics (of the usability assessor):
  - User's gender, which is measured on a nominal scale with two values (male/female)
  - User's computer experience, which is measured on a ratio scale (years)
  - User's Web experience, which is measured on a ratio scale (years)
  - User's computer usage frequency, which is measured on a ratio scale (hours per week)
  - User's Web usage frequency, which is measured on a ratio scale (hours per week)
- User's Internet connection speed, which can be divided into two nominal groups: slow connection (dial-up modem) and fast connection (broadband cable/DSL)

- Purpose of Web site, which is measured on a nominal scale with three possible values: information, entertainment, e-commerce

There were multiple steps involved in the data analysis of the Phase One experiment as follows:

1. Raw usability scores from the respondents were normalised, when necessary, by inverting Likert point of unfavourable[10] statements (5 to 1, 4 to 2, 2 to 4, 1 to 5).
2. For each Web site, the mean of the normalised usability scores was calculated to form *Site Usability Score*.
3. Site Usability Scores of Flash and HTML versions of each Web site were compared using independent t-test to find if there was any significant difference between the usability of Flash and HTML versions of particular Web sites. The combined case of all Web sites was also considered and corresponding t-tests were performed.
4. Multiple independent t-tests and two-way ANOVA (Analysis of Variance) tests were utilised to find if user's characteristics, Internet connection speed, or Web site purpose (in addition to Flash/HTML implementation), could affect Site Usability Scores.

The results of this quantitative analysis were also augmented by analysis of the qualitative data (participant comments). Further discussion regarding the analysis of this experiment and corresponding results is presented in Chapter 8. A review of all data and results of this experiment was used to identify the key issues relating to the research hypotheses which needed further study; this influenced the design of Phase Two.

7.6 Experimental Design for the Phase Two Experiment (Eye Gaze Tracking)

In this phase, an eye gaze tracking experiment was conducted with 39 participants, all of whom were undergraduate students in Murdoch University studying a Human-Computer Interaction unit of study at the time of the experiment. All of the students had participated in the Phase One experiment (online survey). Similar to the survey, participants were separated into two groups: (1) Group A (19 participants) was asked to visit the Flash version of the Web sites; and (2) Group B (20 participants) was asked to visit the HTML version. The grouping was made so that each participant was required to visit the opposite version to what they did in the Phase One experiment. The justification for this rule is that after the participants had completed both online survey and eye gaze tracking experiment, they would have already been familiar with both Flash and HTML versions of the Web sites. Therefore, they were able to rate their personal preferences for each Web site in a post-test questionnaire.

---

[10] The questionnaires included some questions phrased positively and some negatively. Hence, some of the raw scores had to be inverted so that a low value always indicated poor usability.

Although six Web sites were used in the Phase One experiment, only three Web sites were selected for the Phase Two experiment to keep the duration within reasonable limits, as the eye gaze tracking process took considerably longer time than the survey used in the Phase One experiment. These three Web sites were chosen from those used in the Phase One experiment, and the selection was made so that one Web site was chosen from each of the three categories (information, entertainment, e-commerce). The three Web sites selected were:

1. Full Sail (information site)
2. Madonna (entertainment site)
3. Chronicle Books (e-commerce site)

These Web sites were chosen because the results of the Phase One experiment suggested that these three sites provided a higher level of significance (for the experimental variables) than the other Web site within each category, when comparing the usability of Flash and HTML versions.

The eye gaze tracking experiment was conducted in a specialised laboratory located within the Murdoch University campus. The laboratory was equipped with Seeing Machines' faceLAB 3.2.1 head/eye tracking system (the latest version at the time of the experiment), which included faceLAB PC (for running the tracking software), Stereo-Head (dual cameras for capturing face/eye images), and the Overlay Unit. The installation of the faceLAB system was completed one week prior to the experiment. In addition to the faceLAB PC, another PC with a 17-inch monitor (User PC) was used to display Web sites to the user during the experiment. While eye gaze tracking was in process, faceLAB PC also generated Screen Intersections that displayed the approximate area on the screen where the user was looking at, represented as a red dot on the screen. Screen Intersections were also shown to the user during the screen calibration process, just before the start of the experiment. During screen calibration, a white dot appeared on the screen and moved to different points around the screen. The user was required to stare directly at the white dot, so that the cameras could capture images of the user's eyes when he/she looked at different parts of the screen. When the screen calibration finished, the user could no longer see Screen Intersections. Instead, he/she was presented with stimulators (Web sites). However, both Screen Intersections and Web sites were visible to the experimenter at all times. They were also combined (using the Overlay Unit), and then recorded for future analyses. The following schematic diagram depicts the connection of all equipment within the laboratory. Additional images of the laboratory can be found in Appendix 7E.

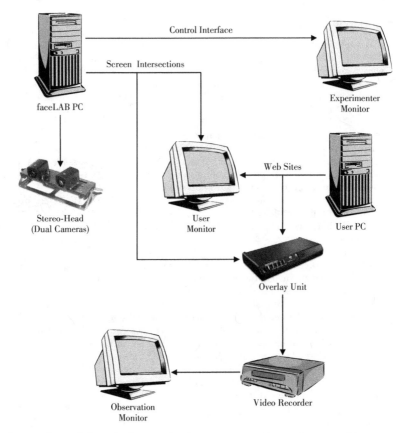

Figure 7.1   Schematic diagram showing eye gaze tracking equipment and its connection

During the two-week experimental period, each of the participants visited the eye tracking laboratory one by one. Each participant was given a one-hour time slot for the experiment, and he/she was monitored by the researcher who was also present in the laboratory while the experiment was taking place. When entering the room, the participant was asked to put four markers on their face (as shown in Figure 7.2) and sit on an adjustable chair in front of the cameras and PC monitor.

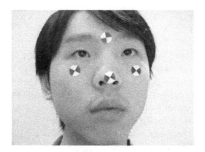

Figure 7.2   Positions of four markers on the user's face

Markers were used on all participants (except one participant who was allergic to Latex material used in the markers) because they were recommended by Seeing Machines for increasing tracking accuracy. After the user applied the markers and adjusted the height of the chair, their face model was created as per faceLAB guidelines, and then eye gaze calibration and screen calibration took place. Detailed procedures for the user and experimenter can be found in Appendix 7F and 7G, respectively.

After the screen calibration, the participant was asked to view a brief PowerPoint presentation on the screen to measure the accuracy of the tracking process. The presentation displayed multiple five-digit numbers on the screen, one by one, on different parts of the screen, and the user was asked to read the numbers out loud in order to aid the experimenter in verifying the accuracy of eye gaze tracking. When the presentation finished, the user was directed (via an onscreen message) to a Web page where they could select the Flash or HTML version (according to their group) and then they were presented with links to the corresponding version of the three Web sites mentioned earlier. The user then followed use scenarios for each Web site (Appendix 7H). While the participant was browsing the Web sites, their eye movement data was collected automatically by the faceLAB system. When they finished, the user was presented with a brief questionnaire asking for their personal preference for each web site. The following choices were available:

- Flash version is a lot better
- Flash version is a little bit better
- Both versions are equally good
- HTML version is a little bit better
- HTML version is a lot better

On the same screen, links to both Flash and HTML versions of each web site were also provided, so that the user could revisit them if they needed to.

7.7 Conclusion

In this chapter, detailed procedures regarding the design and implementation of the Phase One experiment (WUCET usability survey) and the Phase Two experiment (eye gaze tracking) have been examined with respect to the research hypotheses previously discussed. In the following two chapters (Chapter 8 and Chapter 9), the analysis of Phase One and Phase Two experiments and their results will be discussed in detail. In addition, findings and conclusions of the entire research study, together with recommendations for further research, will be discussed in the final chapter of this book (Chapter 10).

8

Results of the Phase One Experiment (Usability Survey)

8.1 Introduction

This chapter reports the results of the first experiment, which involved participants assessing the usability of a set of Web sites. Responses were provided via an online survey. For details of the experimental procedure, see Chapter 7.

There were a total of 43 students who responded to the survey, 20 of whom were randomly selected to view the Flash version of six Web sites, while the rest (23) were assigned to view the HTML version of the same set of Web sites. The number of participants in both groups differs a little because there were a few dropouts during the experiment. However, the difference in numbers is so small that it can be safely ignored. Tables 8.1 and 8.2 depict summaries of the demographic information supplied by the participants.

Table 8.1   Descriptive statistics of participants' demography

Variable	Number of Responses	Minimum	Maximum	Mean	Std. Deviation
Age	43	19	37	23.23	4.810
Computer experience (years)	43	4	21	10.41	3.974
Web experience (years)	43	4	16	6.94	2.366
Computer usage (hours/week)	43	7	80	32.19	17.567
Web usage (hours/week)	43	3	50	17.57	12.741

Table 8.2   Descriptive statistics of participants' demography (continued)

Variable		Frequency	Percentage
Group	Flash	20	46.5
	HTML	23	53.5
Gender	Female	17	39.5
	Male	26	60.5
Internet speed	Slow (56k)	20	46.5
	Medium (64k-128k)	1	2.3
	Fast (≥256k)	21	48.8
	Don't know	1	2.3

8.2   Quantitative Analysis

In this section, each research question and hypothesis proposed in Chapter 6 is re-presented one by one and tested according to quantitative data collected from the Phase One experiment. A summary is given for each hypothesis suggesting whether it is supported or not supported. The significance level of .10 is used as a standard throughout this section because the nature of exploratory research as in this study allows a more lenient level than that of confirmatory research (Garson, 2005; Weisberg, 2002). In essence, it is inappropriate to set a stringent significance level in exploratory research because doing so could limit the possibility of revealing some relationships that really exist and therefore can be confirmed more rigorously by further studies. However, the significance level of .05 or .01 is also presented when available for comparison.

Q1: Is there is a difference in usability of the Flash and HTML versions of a Web site?

H1: The Flash version of a Web site provides higher usability than the HTML version.

In this experiment, the usability of Web sites was measured by the usability score obtained from the WUCET questionnaire (via a Likert scale), presented as real numbers ranging from 1 (least usable) to 5 (most usable). Table 8.3 shows descriptive statistics of the usability score for each Web site (i.e. mean of scores for each usability question for that Web site).

Table 8.3   Descriptive statistics of usability score

Web Site	Version	Number of Responses	Mean Usability Score	Std. Deviation	Std. Error Mean	Mean Difference (Flash-HTML)
A	Flash	20	3.5357	.39777	.08894	.17340
A	HTML	23	3.3623	.38438	.08015	.17340
B	Flash	20	3.6275	.37609	.08410	-.06815
B	HTML	23	3.6957	.39136	.08160	-.06815
C	Flash	20	3.1550	.38726	.08659	.20935
C	HTML	23	2.9457	.44311	.09239	.20935
D	Flash	20	3.4725	.35447	.07926	.23120
D	HTML	23	3.2413	.43502	.09071	.23120
E	Flash	20	3.6250	.38200	.08542	.17500
E	HTML	23	3.4500	.50340	.10497	.17500
F	Flash	20	3.4550	.35685	.07979	.12239
F	HTML	23	3.3326	.42362	.08833	.12239

The graph of mean usability score, grouped by site version, is shown in Figure 8.1.

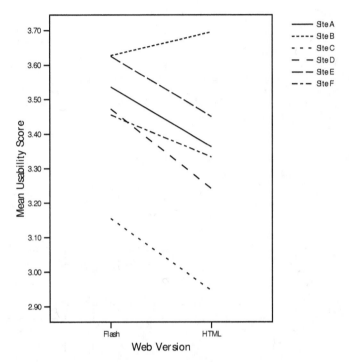

Figure 8.1   Graph of mean usability score of each Web site grouped by site version

According to descriptive statistics (Table 8.3) and graph (Figure 8.1), we can see that five out of six Web sites in the experiment have the Flash version rated higher in usability than the HTML version. For these five Web sites there was a reasonably consistently higher usability rating (by about 0.2 out of 5).

In order to test hypothesis H1, multiple independent t-tests were conducted to compare the mean usability score of Flash version versus HTML version of each Web site. Results from the tests are summarised in Table 8.4.

Table 8.4   Results from independent t-tests comparing mean usability score of
Flash and HTML versions

Web Site	Equal Variances	t	df	Sig. (1-tailed)	Mean Difference	Std. Error Difference
A	assumed	1.452	41	.077*	.17340	.11944
	not assumed	1.448	39.749	.0775*	.17340	.11973
B	assumed	-.580	41	.2825	-.06815	.11751
	not assumed	-.582	40.565	.282	-.06815	.11718
C	assumed	1.637	41	.0545*	.20935	.12785
	not assumed	1.653	40.997	.053*	.20935	.12663
D	assumed	1.892	41	.033**	.23120	.12221
	not assumed	1.919	40.848	.031**	.23120	.12046
E	assumed	1.269	41	.106	.17500	.13796
	not assumed	1.293	40.315	.1015	.17500	.13533
F	assumed	1.016	41	.158	.12239	.12049
	not assumed	1.028	40.967	.155	.12239	.11904

* = significant at .10, ** = significant at .05

From the table, independent t-test results suggest that H1 be supported for Web site
A, C, and D at .10 significance level. However, at .05 significance level, the results
suggest that H1 be supported for Web site D only.

The analysis of individual Web sites is lacking power because of the high
standard deviation resulting from the nature of the usability constructs and the low
number of participants. Therefore, it is more useful to look at the combined situation
(combining responses for each version of Web site, over all Web sites), where the
number of cases increases to 258 (the product of 43 participants and six Web sites).
Tables 8.5 and 8.6 show descriptive statistics and independent t-test results of this
combined situation.

Table 8.5   Descriptive statistics of usability score (combined situation)

Version	Number of Responses	Mean Usability Score	Std. Deviation	Std. Error Mean	Mean Difference (Flash-HTML)
Flash	120	3.4785	.40132	.03664	.14053
HTML	138	3.3379	.48047	.04090	

Table 8.6   Results from independent t-test comparing mean usability score of Flash and HTML Web sites (combined situation)

Equal Variances	t	df	Sig. (1-tailed)	Mean Difference	Std. Error Difference
assumed	2.528	256	.006***	.14053	.05560
not assumed	2.559	255.602	.0055***	.14053	.05491

*** = significant at .01

From Table 8.6, it is suggested that Flash Web sites provide a higher usability score than HTML Web sites at a significance level as low as .01. This can be seen as a generalisation of hypothesis H1, i.e. Flash versions of Web sites (in general) provide higher usability than HTML versions of Web sites.

Q2: Does users' gender affect their perception of the comparative usability of the Flash vs. HTML versions of a Web site?

H2: Male users prefer the Flash version of a Web site (over the HTML version) to a greater extent than do female users.

First, descriptive statistics of usability score, categorised by users' gender, were produced, as shown in Table 8.7. Corresponding graphs are displayed in Figures 8.2 and 8.3 for female and male participants, respectively.

Table 8.7 Descriptive statistics of usability score (grouped by users' gender)

Gender	Web Site	Version	Number of Responses	Mean Usability Score	Std. Deviation	Std. Error Mean	Mean Difference (Flash-HTML)
Female	A	Flash	7	3.5034	.39732	.15017	.15102
		HTML	10	3.3524	.33083	.10462	
	B	Flash	7	3.4429	.40766	.15408	-.25714
		HTML	10	3.7000	.28382	.08975	
	C	Flash	7	3.0786	.35102	.13267	-.05143
		HTML	10	3.1300	.53707	.16984	
	D	Flash	7	3.4929	.15392	.05818	.21786
		HTML	10	3.2750	.44488	.14068	
	E	Flash	7	3.5714	.27667	.10457	.12643
		HTML	10	3.4450	.51556	.16304	
	F	Flash	7	3.4214	.39566	.14955	.29143
		HTML	10	3.1300	.31198	.09866	
Male	A	Flash	13	3.5531	.41310	.11457	.18315
		HTML	13	3.3700	.43433	.12046	
	B	Flash	13	3.7269	.33205	.09209	.03462
		HTML	13	3.6923	.46942	.13019	
	C	Flash	13	3.1962	.41305	.11456	.39231
		HTML	13	2.8038	.30582	.08482	
	D	Flash	13	3.4615	.43212	.11985	.24615
		HTML	13	3.2154	.44365	.12305	
	E	Flash	13	3.6538	.43611	.12096	.20000
		HTML	13	3.4538	.51497	.14283	
	F	Flash	13	3.4731	.34977	.09701	-.01538
		HTML	13	3.4885	.44213	.12263	

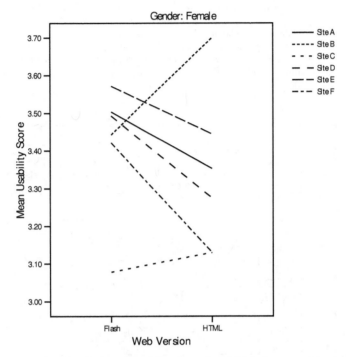

Figure 8.2 Graph of mean usability score of each Web site grouped by site version (female users)

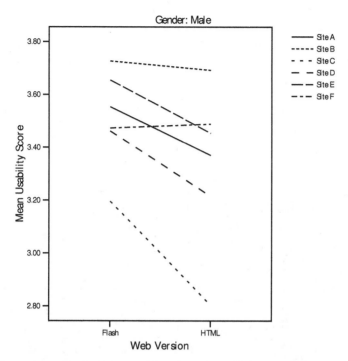

Figure 8.3   Graph of mean usability score of each Web site grouped by site version (male users)

A visual inspection of Figures 8.2 and 8.3 indicates that males appear to rate Flash sites higher in usability (than HTML sites) more consistently than females. Independent t-tests were also performed to compare the usability of Flash and HTML versions of the Web sites, in the same fashion as Table 8.4; however, this time responses were grouped by users' gender before the tests were performed. Results of these tests are shown in Tables 8.8 and 8.9 for female and male participants, respectively.

Table 8.8   Results from independent t-tests comparing mean usability score of Flash and HTML versions (female users)

Web Site	Equal Variances	t	df	Sig. (1-tailed)	Mean Difference	Std. Error Difference
A	assumed	.854	15	.2035	.15102	.17687
	not assumed	.825	11.440	.213	.15102	.18302
B	assumed	-1.540	15	.072*	-.25714	.16698
	not assumed	-1.442	9.995	.09*	-.25714	.17832
C	assumed	-.221	15	.414	-.05143	.23238
	not assumed	-.239	14.972	.4075	-.05143	.21551
D	assumed	1.235	15	.118	.21786	.17647
	not assumed	1.431	11.823	.089*	.21786	.15224
E	assumed	.588	15	.2825	.12643	.21487
	not assumed	.653	14.298	.262	.12643	.19369
F	assumed	1.700	15	.055*	.29143	.17144
	not assumed	1.627	10.973	.066*	.29143	.17916

* = significant at .10

From Table 8.8, it can be seen that for female participants, the Flash version of Web sites D and F produced significantly higher usability score than the HTML version (at the .10 level). It is worth noticing that for Web site D, equal variances are not assumed because the p value of Lavene's test for equality of variances is .033 (less than .05). For Web site B, the HTML version was rated more highly than the Flash version (significant at .10 level) by the females.

Table 8.9   Results from independent t-tests comparing mean usability score of Flash and HTML versions (male users)

Web Site	Equal Variances	t	df	Sig. (1-tailed)	Mean Difference	Std. Error Difference
A	assumed	1.102	24	.141	.18315	.16625
	not assumed	1.102	23.940	.141	.18315	.16625
B	assumed	.217	24	.415	.03462	.15947
	not assumed	.217	21.604	.415	.03462	.15947
C	assumed	2.752	24	.0055***	.39231	.14254
	not assumed	2.752	22.116	.006***	.39231	.14254
D	assumed	1.433	24	.0825*	.24615	.17177
	not assumed	1.433	23.983	.0825*	.24615	.17177
E	assumed	1.069	24	.148	.20000	.18716
	not assumed	1.069	23.366	.148	.20000	.18716
F	assumed	-.098	24	.461	-.01538	.15636
	not assumed	-.098	22.793	.461	-.01538	.15636

* = significant at .10, *** = significant at .01

Table 8.9 shows that, for male participants, there are significant differences in the usability score of Flash and HTML versions of Web sites C and D (Flash version received higher score) at .01 and .10 significant levels, respectively.

     For the combined situation, descriptive statistics and t-test results are shown in Tables 8.10 and 8.11.

Table 8.10 Descriptive statistics of usability score (combined situation, grouped by users' gender)

Gender	Version	Number of Responses	Mean Usability Score	Std. Deviation	Std. Error Mean	Mean Difference (Flash-HTML)
Female	Flash	42	3.4184	.35921	.05543	.07969
	HTML	60	3.3387	.44508	.05746	
Male	Flash	78	3.5108	.42093	.04766	.17347
	HTML	78	3.3373	.50887	.05762	

Table 8.11 Results from independent t-tests comparing mean usability score of Flash and HTML Web sites (combined situation, grouped by users' gender)

Gender	Equal Variances	t	df	Sig. (1-tailed)	Mean Difference	Std. Error Difference
Female	assumed	.961	100	.1695	.07969	.08290
	not assumed	.998	97.902	.1605	.07969	.07984
Male	assumed	2.320	154	.011**	.17347	.07478
	not assumed	2.320	148.771	.011**	.17347	.07478

** = significant at .05

Table 8.11 shows that there is a significant difference in Web site usability perception patterns of male and female users. Female users see no significant difference in usability between Flash and HTML Web sites (in general), while male users tend to prefer Flash than HTML Web sites, which can be seen as support for the general interpretation of hypothesis H2.

However, in order to test hypothesis H2 in a stricter sense (where the Flash version of a Web site is compared to the HTML version of that Web site only), two variables were selected as independent variables: (1) version of Web site visited (Flash/HTML); and (2) gender (female/male). The dependent variable is usability score from WUCET questionnaire. Multiple plots were created to see if there is any effect of both independent variables on usability score of each Web site, as shown in Figures 8.4-8.6.

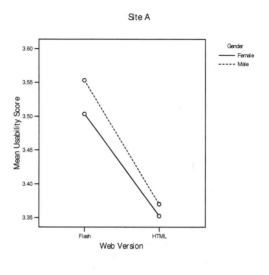

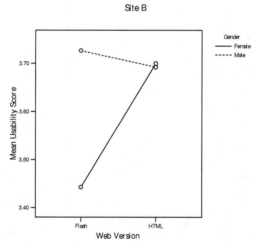

Figure 8.4   Plots of usability score as dependent on site version and users'
gender (Web sites A and B)

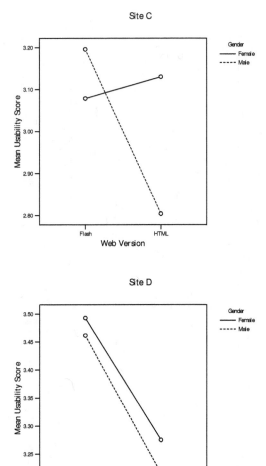

Figure 8.5 Plots of usability score as dependent on site version and users' gender (Web sites C and D)

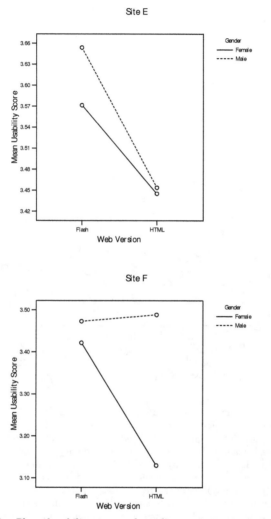

Figure 8.6   Plots of usability score as dependent on site version and users'
gender (Web sites E and F)

The plots depicted in Figures 8.4-8.6 suggest that male users prefer the Flash
version while female users prefer the HTML version in Web sites B and C; and

female users prefer the Flash version while male users prefer the HTML version in Web site F. For other Web sites, both gender groups prefer the Flash version to the HTML version.

In order to test this hypothesis quantitatively, two-way ANOVA (analysis of variance) was used. Table 8.12 summarises the results from multiple ANOVA tests.

Table 8.12 ANOVA test results for hypothesis H2

Source	Web Site	Type III Sum of Squares	df	Mean Square	F	Sig.
Version	A	.281	1	.281	1.758	.193
	B	.125	1	.125	.856	.361
	C	.293	1	.293	1.756	.193
	D	.543	1	.543	3.243	.079
	E	.269	1	.269	1.260	.269
	F	.192	1	.192	1.331	.256
Gender	A	.011	1	.011	.071	.791
	B	.193	1	.193	1.320	.258
	C	.110	1	.110	.657	.422
	D	.021	1	.021	.125	.726
	E	.021	1	.021	.098	.755
	F	.424	1	.424	2.937	.094
Version * Gender	A	.003	1	.003	.016	.899
	B	.215	1	.215	1.471	.233
	C	.496	1	.496	2.976	.092
	D	.002	1	.002	.012	.913
	E	.014	1	.014	.064	.802
	F	.237	1	.237	1.644	.207

The significance values in Table 8.12 show that for the majority of Web sites (A, C, D, E), the Web site version has more significant effect on usability score than users' gender, thus supporting the results found in the equivalent t-tests performed previously for hypothesis H1. However, when considering both factors (site version and gender) at the same time, only one Web site (C) shows significance at .10 level. Therefore, the concurrent effect of site version and gender cannot be asserted quantitatively, even though visual representation may suggest so. It also follows that H2 is not supported for the separate analysis of each Web site (in contrast to the combined analysis where H2 was supported). The number of participants may need to be significantly increased to demonstrate a significant effect of gender on each individual Web site.

Q3:   Does users' computer/Web experience affect their perception of the comparative usability of the Flash vs. HTML versions of a Web site?

H3:   Users with shorter computer/Web experience prefer the Flash version of a Web site (over the HTML version) to a greater extent than do users with longer computer/Web experience.

In order to measure computer/Web experience of the users, a new variable was created using the following formula:

$$\text{Combined experience} = \text{Computer experience (years)} \times \text{Computer usage (hours/week)} + \text{Web experience (years)} \times \text{Web usage (hours/week)}$$

A median was computed for this variable (median=370), then users were grouped into two categories—those with combined experience below 370 were grouped as having "short-term" computer/Web experience, while the rest were grouped as having "long-term" computer/Web experience. Table 8.13 depicts descriptive statistics of usability score, grouped by users' experience. Corresponding graphs are shown in Figures 8.7 and 8.8.

Table 8.13 Descriptive statistics of usability score (grouped by users' experience)

Experience	Web Site	Version	N	Mean Usability Score	Std. Deviation	Std. Error Mean	Mean Difference (Flash-HTML)
Long-term	A	Flash	8	3.3750	.40039	.14156	.04507
		HTML	14	3.3299	.39992	.10688	
	B	Flash	8	3.7563	.28339	.10020	.07411
		HTML	14	3.6821	.37345	.09981	
	C	Flash	8	3.1313	.40438	.14297	.07054
		HTML	14	3.0607	.42070	.11244	
	D	Flash	8	3.3937	.51785	.18309	.28661
		HTML	14	3.1071	.36996	.09888	
	E	Flash	8	3.6188	.49637	.17549	.13661
		HTML	14	3.4821	.55109	.14728	
	F	Flash	8	3.4813	.28023	.09907	.07054
		HTML	14	3.4107	.40770	.10896	
Short-term	A	Flash	12	3.6429	.37413	.10800	.23016
		HTML	9	3.4127	.37646	.12549	
	B	Flash	12	3.5417	.41606	.12011	-.17500
		HTML	9	3.7167	.44017	.14672	
	C	Flash	12	3.1708	.39281	.11339	.40417
		HTML	9	2.7667	.43946	.14649	
	D	Flash	12	3.5250	.19714	.05691	.07500
		HTML	9	3.4500	.46637	.15546	
	E	Flash	12	3.6292	.30856	.08907	.22917
		HTML	9	3.4000	.44581	.14860	
	F	Flash	12	3.4375	.41128	.11873	.22639
		HTML	9	3.2111	.44284	.14761	

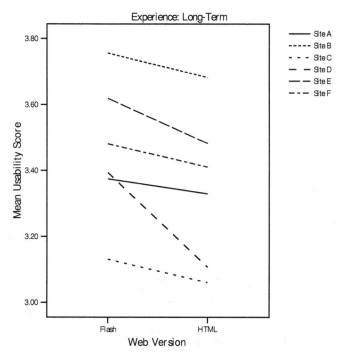

Figure 8.7   Graph of mean usability score of each Web site grouped by site
version (long-term users)

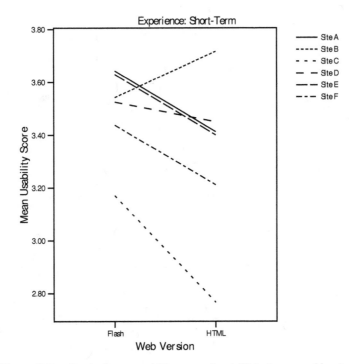

Figure 8.8   Graph of mean usability score of each Web site grouped by site version (short-term users)

In similar fashion to the analysis of hypothesis H2, independent t-tests were performed for each Web site, after the responses were separated into two experience groups. The results of the tests are presented in Tables 8.14 and 8.15 for users with long-term and short-term experience, respectively.

Table 8.14 Results from independent t-tests comparing mean usability score of Flash and HTML versions (long-term users)

Web Site	Equal Variances	t	df	Sig. (1-tailed)	Mean Difference	Std. Error Difference
A	assumed	.254	20	.401	.04507	.17732
	not assumed	.254	14.686	.4015	.04507	.17738
B	assumed	.485	20	.3165	.07411	.15274
	not assumed	.524	18.158	.3035	.07411	.14142
C	assumed	.383	20	.3525	.07054	.18396
	not assumed	.388	15.205	.352	.07054	.18189
D	assumed	1.512	20	.073*	.28661	.18950
	not assumed	1.377	11.167	.0975*	.28661	.20808
E	assumed	.579	20	.2845	.13661	.23604
	not assumed	.596	16.047	.2795	.13661	.22911
F	assumed	.432	20	.335	.07054	.16316
	not assumed	.479	19.116	.3185	.07054	.14727

* = significant at .10

Table 8.14 suggests that for users who have long-term experience with computers and the Web, only one Web site (site D) shows significant difference in usability between its Flash and HTML versions. For all other Web sites, the difference is not significant at .10 level.

Table 8.15 Results from independent t-tests comparing mean usability score of Flash and HTML versions (short-term users)

Web Site	Equal Variances	t	df	Sig. (1-tailed)	Mean Difference	Std. Error Difference
A	assumed	1.391	19	.09*	.23016	.16541
	not assumed	1.390	17.327	.091*	.23016	.16556
B	assumed	-.931	19	.182	-.17500	.18802
	not assumed	-.923	16.821	.1845	-.17500	.18961
C	assumed	2.219	19	.0195**	.40417	.18216
	not assumed	2.182	16.223	.022**	.40417	.18525
D	assumed	.504	19	.31	.07500	.14894
	not assumed	.453	10.155	.33	.07500	.16555
E	assumed	1.395	19	.0895*	.22917	.16429
	not assumed	1.323	13.513	.104	.22917	.17326
F	assumed	1.208	19	.121	.22639	.18734
	not assumed	1.195	16.635	.1245	.22639	.18944

* = significant at .10, ** = significant at .05

Independent t-test results in Table 8.15 show that for users with short-term experience, Web sites A, C, and E produced significant differences in the usability of their Flash and HTML versions (Flash version was rated higher). For Web site E, equal variances are assumed because the p value of Lavene's test is .462 (higher than .05).

For the combined situation, descriptive statistics and t-test results are summarised in Tables 8.16 and 8.17.

Table 8.16 Descriptive statistics of usability score (combined situation, grouped by users' experience)

Experience	Version	Number of Responses	Mean Usability Score	Std. Deviation	Std. Error Mean	Mean Difference (Flash-HTML)
Long-term	Flash	48	3.4594	.43382	.06262	.11391
	HTML	84	3.3455	.46469	.05070	
Short-term	Flash	72	3.4912	.38072	.04487	.16498
	HTML	54	3.3262	.50825	.06916	

Table 8.17 Results from independent t-tests comparing mean usability score of Flash and HTML Web sites (combined situation, grouped by users' experience)

Experience	Equal Variances	t	df	Sig. (1-tailed)	Mean Difference	Std. Error Difference
Long-term	assumed	1.387	130	.084*	.11391	.08210
	not assumed	1.414	103.614	.08*	.11391	.08057
Short-term	assumed	2.084	124	.0195**	.16498	.07917
	not assumed	2.001	94.502	.024**	.16498	.08244

* = significant at .10, ** = significant at .05

In the analysis of the combined situation, both groups show a significance difference in usability of Flash and HTML Web sites at the .10 significant level. However, at the .05 significant level, only the short-term experience group shows this difference, which means that users with shorter computer/Web experience prefer the Flash version to a greater extent than long-term users, and therefore, hypothesis H3 is weakly supported in this combined analysis.

In order to test hypothesis H3 separately for each Web site, the plots in Figures 8.9-8.11 were made to show the usability score for each Web site as dependent on site version and users' experience.

Site A

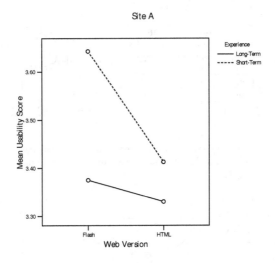

Site B

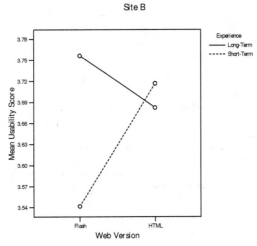

Figure 8.9   Plots of usability score as dependent on site version and users'
computer/Web experience (Web sites A and B)

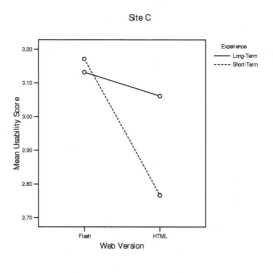

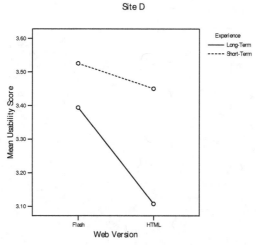

Figure 8.10 Plots of usability score as dependent on site version and users' computer/Web experience (Web sites C and D)

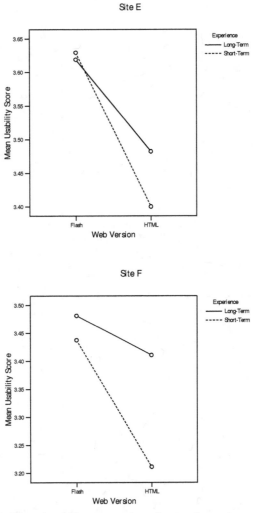

Figure 8.11 Plots of usability score as dependent on site version and users' computer/Web experience (Web sites E and F)

According to the plots in Figures 8.9-8.11, only Web site B shows that long-term users and short-term users have conflicting preferences for the Flash version of the

Web site compared to the HTML version (long-term users prefer the Flash version while short-term users prefer the HTML version). For all other Web sites, both groups prefer the Flash version to the HTML version. ANOVA tests were performed to find the significance of this effect, as shown in Table 8.18.

Table 8.18   ANOVA test results for hypothesis H3

Source	Web Site	Type III Sum of Squares	df	Mean Square	F	Sig.
Version	A	.194	1	.194	1.287	.264
	B	.026	1	.026	.174	.679
	C	.577	1	.577	3.362	.074
	D	.335	1	.335	2.240	.143
	E	.342	1	.342	1.606	.213
	F	.226	1	.226	1.433	.239
Experience	A	.315	1	.315	2.088	.156
	B	.083	1	.083	.555	.461
	C	.166	1	.166	.966	.332
	D	.575	1	.575	3.851	.057
	E	.013	1	.013	.062	.805
	F	.152	1	.152	.962	.333
Version * Experience	A	.088	1	.088	.582	.450
	B	.159	1	.159	1.062	.309
	C	.285	1	.285	1.661	.205
	D	.115	1	.115	.767	.386
	E	.022	1	.022	.103	.750
	F	.062	1	.062	.395	.533

ANOVA results from Table 8.18 show that the usability of each Web site in the experiment does not depend on Web site version viewed by the users and their computer/Web experience at the same time (at any significance level less than .20). Therefore, hypothesis H3 is not supported for the analysis of each Web site individually, due to the small number of responses.

In addition to categorising participants into two experience groups, the computer/Web experience variable can also be treated on a continuum. Scatterplots of experience score and mean rating of usability (all Web sites) for Flash and HTML groups are displayed in Figures 8.12 and 8.13, respectively.

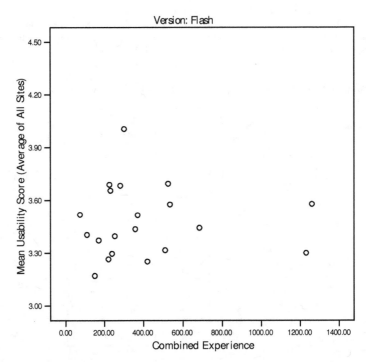

Figure 8.12 Scatterplot of experience score and mean usability rating (Flash group)

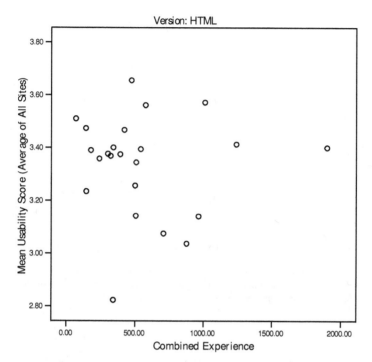

Figure 8.13 Scatterplot of experience score and mean usability rating (HTML group)

The scatterplot in Figure 8.12 shows that users with less experience tend to rate the Flash sites higher in usability than users with more experience. On the other hand, Figure 8.13 shows that users with less experience tend to rate the HTML sites lower in usability than users with more experience. However, the effect is so subtle that Pearson's correlation does not show any significant result (Flash: $r = -.007$, $p = .977$; HTML: $r = -.028$, $p = .898$).

Q4: Does users' Internet connection speed affect their perception of the comparative usability of the Flash vs. HTML versions of a Web site?

H4: Users with slower Internet connection speed see the difference in usability between the Flash and HTML versions of a Web site to a greater extent than do users with faster Internet connection speed.

Users' Internet connection speed was first categorised into three groups: slow (56k, e.g. dial-up), medium (64k-128k, e.g. ISDN), and fast (≥256k, e.g. DSL, cable, T1). However, only one participant responded that he/she used a medium speed connection, so it is more appropriate to consider only two groups (slow/fast) for statistical analysis of hypothesis H4. Therefore, two participants were omitted from this analysis, one is the person with medium speed connection as mentioned earlier, the other person stated that he/she did not know what the speed of his/her Internet connection was.

The analysis was done with many similar aspects to hypothesis H2 and H3. However, the difference is that for H2 and H3, one-tailed t-tests were utilised because it was hypothesised that the Flash version would be rated higher in usability, while in the case of H4, it was still unknown whether the Flash or HTML version would be preferred (since Flash Web sites tend to load more slowly at first, but after fully loaded, could be browsed faster because many parts of the site have already been loaded, while HTML sites can only be loaded one page at a time).

First, descriptive statistics were produced as shown in Table 8.19. Corresponding plots are displayed in Figures 8.14 and 8.15 for users with slow and fast Internet connection, respectively.

Table 8.19 Descriptive statistics of usability score (grouped by users' experience)

Speed	Web Site	Version	N	Mean Usability Score	Std. Deviation	Std. Error Mean	Mean Difference (Flash-HTML)
Slow	A	Flash	6	3.5397	.45142	.18429	.24376
		HTML	14	3.2959	.39717	.10615	
	B	Flash	6	3.9000	.37815	.15438	.17143
		HTML	14	3.7286	.40322	.10776	
	C	Flash	6	3.3750	.41563	.16968	.50357
		HTML	14	2.8714	.40274	.10764	
	D	Flash	6	3.3917	.30069	.12276	.15238
		HTML	14	3.2393	.45875	.12261	
	E	Flash	6	3.5917	.36113	.14743	.21667
		HTML	14	3.3750	.53196	.14217	
	F	Flash	6	3.7417	.35835	.14630	.55952
		HTML	14	3.1821	.33833	.09042	
Fast	A	Flash	13	3.5421	.40571	.11252	.04212
		HTML	8	3.5000	.36973	.13072	
	B	Flash	13	3.5077	.33345	.09248	-.17356
		HTML	8	3.6813	.39994	.14140	
	C	Flash	13	3.0538	.36082	.10007	.08510
		HTML	8	2.9688	.44716	.15810	
	D	Flash	13	3.5115	.39537	.10965	.31779
		HTML	8	3.1938	.42125	.14894	
	E	Flash	13	3.6308	.41810	.11596	.08702
		HTML	8	3.5438	.48656	.17203	
	F	Flash	13	3.3538	.28684	.07955	-.33365
		HTML	8	3.6875	.29246	.10340	

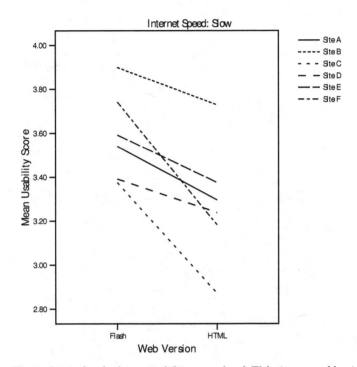

Figure 8.14 Graph of mean usability score of each Web site grouped by site version (users with slow Internet connection)

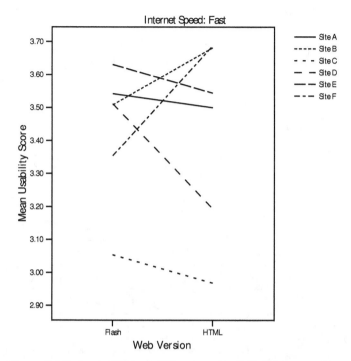

Figure 8.15 Graph of mean usability score of each Web site grouped by site version (users with fast Internet connection)

From Figures 8.14 and 8.15, it can be seen that users with a slow Internet connection have a uniform preference for the Flash version of all Web sites, while users with a faster Internet connection prefer the Flash version of four Web sites and the HTML version of two Web sites. This difference can also be seen on t-test results as shown in Tables 8.20 and 8.21.

Table 8.20   Results from independent t-tests comparing mean usability score of
Flash and HTML versions (users with slow Internet connection)

Web Site	Equal Variances	t	df	Sig. (2-tailed)	Mean Difference	Std. Error Difference
A	assumed	1.210	18	.242	.24376	.20150
	not assumed	1.146	8.508	.283	.24376	.21268
B	assumed	.886	18	.387	.17143	.19343
	not assumed	.911	10.134	.384	.17143	.18827
C	assumed	2.540	18	.021**	.50357	.19828
	not assumed	2.506	9.257	.033**	.50357	.20094
D	assumed	.742	18	.468	.15238	.20535
	not assumed	.878	14.429	.394	.15238	.17350
E	assumed	.905	18	.377	.21667	.23935
	not assumed	1.058	13.975	.308	.21667	.20481
F	assumed	3.333	18	.004***	.55952	.16786
	not assumed	3.253	9.042	.010***	.55952	.17198

** = significant at .05, *** = significant at .01

For users with a slow Internet connection speed, Web sites C and F show a significant difference in usability between the Flash and HTML versions at .05 and .01 significant levels, respectively.

Table 8.21 Results from independent t-tests comparing mean usability score of Flash and HTML versions (users with fast Internet connection)

Web Site	Equal Variances	t	df	Sig. (2-tailed)	Mean Difference	Std. Error Difference
A	assumed	.239	19	.814	.04212	.17653
	not assumed	.244	16.070	.810	.04212	.17248
B	assumed	-1.075	19	.296	-.17356	.16149
	not assumed	-1.027	12.893	.323	-.17356	.16896
C	assumed	.480	19	.637	.08510	.17742
	not assumed	.455	12.557	.657	.08510	.18711
D	assumed	1.746	19	.097*	.31779	.18203
	not assumed	1.718	14.210	.107	.31779	.18495
E	assumed	.436	19	.668	.08702	.19976
	not assumed	.419	13.215	.682	.08702	.20746
F	assumed	-2.570	19	.019**	-.33365	.12983
	not assumed	-2.557	14.729	.022**	-.33365	.13046

* = significant at .10, ** = significant at .05

Regarding users with a fast Internet connection, Web site D shows a significant difference in usability between the Flash and HTML versions (the Flash version was rated higher) at the .10 significant level (equal variances assumed because the significance of Lavene's test is .713), while Web site F shows a significant difference at the .05 level (HTML version was rated higher).

The combined analysis was done in the same fashion as for the previous hypotheses, except that two-tailed t-tests were performed instead of one-tailed. Descriptive statistics and t-test results are displayed in Tables 8.22 and 8.23.

Table 8.22   Descriptive statistics of usability score (combined situation, grouped by users' Internet speed)

Speed	Version	Number of Responses	Mean Usability Score	Std. Deviation	Std. Error Mean	Mean Difference (Flash-HTML)
Slow	Flash	36	3.5899	.39954	.06659	.30789
	HTML	84	3.2821	.48615	.05304	
Fast	Flash	78	3.4333	.40450	.04580	.00414
	HTML	48	3.4292	.46816	.06757	

Table 8.23   Results from independent t-tests comparing mean usability score of Flash and HTML Web sites (combined situation, grouped by users' Internet speed)

Speed	Equal Variances	t	df	Sig. (2-tailed)	Mean Difference	Std. Error Difference
Slow	Assumed	3.344	118	.001***	.30789	.09206
	Not assumed	3.617	79.937	.001***	.30789	.08513
Fast	Assumed	.052	124	.958	.00414	.07884
	Not assumed	.051	88.680	.960	.00414	.08163

*** = significant at .01

The results of t-tests in Tables 8.22 and 8.23 suggest that users with a slow Internet connection speed have a highly significant preference for the Flash version over the HTML version (at a significant level of << .01), while users with a fast Internet connection do not see a significant difference between the Flash and HTML versions. Therefore, hypothesis H4 is supported.

Q5:   Does the category of a Web site (information, entertainment, e-commerce) affect the comparative usability of the Flash vs. HTML versions of the Web site?

H5:   The category of a Web site (information, entertainment, e-commerce) affects the comparative usability of the Flash vs. HTML versions of the Web site.

For hypothesis H5, responses were combined according to Web site purpose/category, i.e. sites A and B were grouped as information sites, sites C and D were grouped as entertainment sites, sites E and F were grouped as e-commerce sites. Table 8.24 shows descriptive statistics of the usability score after this categorisation was made. The corresponding graph is shown in Figure 8.16.

Table 8.24 Descriptive statistics of usability score (grouped by site purpose)

Site Purpose	Version	Number of Responses	Mean Usability Score	Std. Deviation	Std. Error Mean	Mean Difference (Flash-HTML)
E-commerce	Flash	40	3.5400	.37488	.05927	.14870
	HTML	46	3.3913	.46384	.06839	
Entertainment	Flash	40	3.3138	.40016	.06327	.22027
	HTML	46	3.0935	.45918	.06770	
Information	Flash	40	3.5816	.38490	.06086	.05262
	HTML	46	3.5290	.41894	.06177	

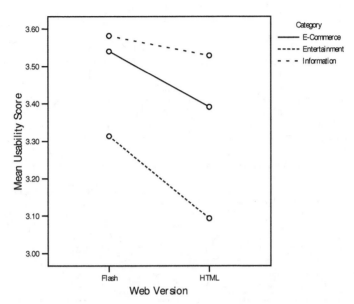

Figure 8.16 Plots of usability score as dependent on site version and category of Web site

It can be inferred from Figure 8.16 that no matter which category a Web site falls into, Flash Web sites were rated higher in usability than HTML Web sites. However, it is worth noticing (from the slope) that the difference in usability of Flash versus HTML Web sites seems to be much greater in entertainment and e-commerce Web sites than information Web sites. This characteristic was as expected because entertainment and e-commerce Web sites tend to contain more multimedia contents (graphics, sounds, etc.) than information Web sites and therefore are more suitable to be implemented in Flash. Table 8.25 summarises the results from corresponding t-tests that show the significance of this difference.

Table 8.25 Results from independent t-tests comparing mean usability score of Flash and HTML Web sites (grouped by site purpose)

Site Purpose	Equal Variances	t	df	Sig. (1-tailed)	Mean Difference	Std. Error Difference
E-commerce	assumed	1.619	84	.0545*	.14870	.09185
	not assumed	1.643	83.581	.052*	.14870	.09050
Entertainment	assumed	2.354	84	.0105**	.22027	.09356
	not assumed	2.377	83.999	.01**	.22027	.09266
Information	assumed	.603	84	.274	.05262	.08723
	not assumed	.607	83.731	.273	.05262	.08671

* = significant at .10, ** = significant at .05

From Table 8.25, it can be seen that for entertainment and e-commerce Web sites, the Flash version is rated significantly higher than the HTML version (at the .05 and .10 significant levels, respectively), while information Web sites show no significant difference in usability of Flash and HTML versions. Therefore, it can be concluded that hypothesis H5 is supported.

Q6: Does the version of a Web site visited (Flash or HTML) affect users' inclination and ability to perform tasks (use scenarios) within Web site, as reflected by the task completion score?

H6: The version of a Web site visited (Flash or HTML) affects users' inclination and ability to perform tasks (use scenarios) within Web site, as reflected by the task completion score.

During the experiment, while participants visited the Web sites, they were also asked to answer five multiple-choice questions per Web site concerning the results of search scenarios, for a total of 30 questions. Each question was given one point (for a correct answer), so the full score was 30 points. Although 43 participants completed the survey, only 41 participants submitted their answers to the multiple-choice questions. Of all 41 participants, 18 visited the Flash version of the Web sites, while the rest (23) visited the HTML version. Four participants missed answering questions for one Web site (mostly because of technical difficulties), so they were given 2.5 as the score of that Web site (because each Web site can have a score ranging from 0 to 5). Table 8.26 depicts descriptive statistics of the score.

Table 8.26 Descriptive statistics of task completion score

Group	Number of Responses	Minimum	Maximum	Mean	Std. Deviation
Flash	18	22.5	29	26.0278	1.68446
HTML	23	19	29	24.6739	3.12107
Total	41	19	29	25.2683	2.65070

From Table 8.26, it can be inferred that the Flash version provided the users with higher task completion score (26.0278 versus 24.6739). In order to verify the significance of this difference, an independent t-test (two-tailed) was performed as shown in Table 8.27. A two-tailed test was chosen because, according to the hypothesis (before the experiment), it was not predicted whether the Flash or the HTML version would generate a higher score.

Table 8.27 Results from independent t-test comparing mean task completion score of Flash and HTML versions

Equal Variances	t	df	Sig. (2-tailed)	Mean Difference	Std. Error Difference
assumed	1.658	39	.105	1.35386	.81650
not assumed	1.776	35.127	.084*	1.35386	.76234

* = significant at .10

From Table 8.27, we can see that the difference in the task completion score of the Flash and HTML versions is significant at the .10 level (equal variances not assumed because Lavene's test significance is .009). Therefore, hypothesis H6 is weakly supported by statistical evidence from the experiment. In addition, we can also conclude that the Flash version of the Web sites provided users with a higher task completion score than the HTML version. However, the effect is weak.

8.3 Qualitative Analysis

Qualitative data was obtained from participants' comments on the six Web sites visited. The participants were given an option whether they wished to provide comments or not, and each participant could comment on any number of Web sites. Table 8.28 summarises the number of participants who provided comments on Flash and HTML versions of each Web site.

Table 8.28   Number of commentary responses for each Web site in the experiment

Web Site	Number of Responses	
	Flash	HTML
A	14	10
B	15	10
C	13	11
D	15	8
E	9	9
F	11	7
Total	77	55
Average	12.83	9.17

It is interesting to see that the average number of commentary responses is 12.83 for Flash Web sites and 9.17 for HTML Web sites, in spite of the lower number of participants in the Flash group (20 participants, compared to 23 participants in the HTML group). This indicates that the Flash versions of the Web sites made users more willing to provide comments than the HTML versions of the Web sites.

In order to analyse the comments provided by the participants qualitatively, preprocessing of comments was performed. First, some comments which contain several ideas (sometimes conflicting) were broken into two or more parts (idea units), each of which contains just one idea that cannot be divided further. Then, each idea unit was classified as representing either positive or negative opinion towards the Web site, and further categorised into four categories: (1) function, (2) design, (3) navigation, and (4) speed. The classification was made in order to assist in identifying explanations for the quantitative results obtained previously. These ideas were also normalised by removing some ideas that were too short, ambiguous, and/or not useful for the analysis (i.e. did not fit the classification schema). Some examples of removed comments include: "Innovative Web site," "Great site," "Really disliked this site," "It was fairly straightforward," and the like. Tables 8.29-8.40 list all the idea units resulting from this categorisation and normalisation process.

Table 8.29   Participants' ideas regarding Web Site A (Flash version)

Polar	Ideas
Positive	*Regarding function:* • The guidance of the man walking you through the site helps a lot. • The introductory animation/speech is great. It makes it both helpful and entertaining, which gives it an attractive first impression. *Regarding design:* • The introduction was quite unique and attractive, specifically when a man comes up and introduces the sites contents in a sophisticated manner. • Very sleek layout, akin to an OS. • The design was attractive.
Negative	*Regarding function:* • At the first look of the website, I did not know what it was for. • The search engine was not that effective as the results did not suit the intended purpose. • The search function wasn't very helpful; it only gave me the information I'd already found myself. *Regarding design:* • The design may be too advanced for novice users on the Internet. • The heading at the top left corner looks too small. • It was a little bit annoying with the flashing images on the home page. • The sound effects became irritating. *Regarding navigation:* • I found the taskbar to be very annoying as it pops up when you place your cursor over it. • I didn't realise that there was a menu button at the bottom of the homepage. This made it difficult for me to navigate at first. • Took a bit of time getting used to navigation. • Difficult to navigate through site - no home button. • It was sometimes different to navigate to find the right information. • It took quite some time to find answers to the questions and I would tend to get lost within the sites' contents. *Regarding speed:* • The website took quite some time to load. • Dial up speeds can affect the amount of time taken to load this Flash site. • Site takes too long to load. • Search system takes too long.

Table 8.30 Participants' ideas regarding Web Site B (Flash version)

Polar	Ideas
Positive	*Regarding function:* • The website had a good introduction. • There was a 'Skip Introduction' option for viewers who may not have time. • It was generally a very informative website. • Its help function was very useful and supportive. • I thought this site was very useful. • Exceedingly concise and very comprehensive. *Regarding design:* • The background colour and the design schemes suited the theme of the army. • This site feels very crisp. • Colour scheme gives it a real 'historic' feel. *Regarding navigation:* • Well laid-out, orange buttons used for more information was useful for me. • I was able to navigate the site easily • The timeline design makes it easy to navigate and gives a good overall summary of past events.
Negative	*Regarding function:* • It was a bit confusing on how to use it. *Regarding navigation:* • Navigation took a bit of getting used to. • There are some small orange colour buttons without labeling, too hard to know where it links to. • It took a couple of minutes to get used to the navigation on this Flash site. • Someone with less experience might have trouble navigating the site. • The yellow bullets were quite annoying because they were placed anywhere and they don't look like they lead to any links. • The movement and transition of the timeline made me feel uneasy and dizzy. • I find the scrolling of the time-line irritating. • I am overwhelmed by the number of hotspots. • Pressing the 'back' button resets the homepage and doesn't go back to the content you chose.

Table 8.31 Participants' ideas regarding Web Site C (Flash version)

Polar	Ideas
Positive	*Regarding function:* • It's clear and concise. *Regarding speed:* • Site is quick loading.
Negative	*Regarding design:* • It was so hard to read, not only was the font faint, but it was extremely small as well. • Sometimes it was annoying with the flashing images. • The words are too small to read on some pages. • The font is tiny and hard to read. • The text was way too small. • Hard to read, i.e. text size and colour.

Table 8.32 Participants' ideas regarding Web Site D (Flash version)

Polar	Ideas
Positive	*Regarding function:* • The special features such as the jukebox, subscription features, and photo gallery suited the theme and promoted the artist well. *Regarding design:* • The website was attractive and suited the theme well. *Regarding navigation:* • The main menu is easy to use. The menu items are located in logical places.
Negative	*Regarding function:* • Broken links would tend to leave a bad impression on viewers and they may tend to exit the website. *Regarding design:* • A bit too much flashing images. *Regarding navigation:* • The scrolling is very slow which annoyed me. • No scrollbars to navigate text. This can be frustrating. *Regarding speed:* • This site takes too much time to load for my computer. • Took forever for each page to load. • Too chunky on my machine, keeps having to load when clicking on another page. • It took a while to load some of the section of the site. Definitely a site which prefers broadband connection. • Took ages to load on my machine. • Far too long for loading. • It was an excruciating wait for the media to load. • The only problem with this site is download speed - it is no good for a 56kps connection, too slow. • It took a while to load each page.

Table 8.33   Participants' ideas regarding Web Site E (Flash version)

Polar	Ideas
Positive	*Regarding function:* • The information on the site was easy to find. • The website had efficient search facilities. • The shopping cart was a good feature that accommodated online payments. • Found it extremely easy to use, liked the site a lot. • This site was useful and good. *Regarding design:* • The website had effective design and colour schemes that suited the topic well. It created a relaxed atmosphere for viewing.
Negative	*Regarding navigation:* • The navigation bar had a few flaws. *Regarding speed:* • Always have problems loading the page. Too slow. • May take while to perform a search. • Sometimes it took a while to get the results after clicking on a link. • The gift finder search took too long and made me lose my patience.

Table 8.34   Participants' ideas regarding Web Site F (Flash version)

Polar	Ideas
Positive	*Regarding function:* • This website is relatively simple and easy to use. • There is good and effective categorisation of information, making it easy to find information. • Simple and easy to use. No hesitation when surfing it. • Very easy to use and obtain the necessary information. • Very clean, concise and simple. Information is where I expect it to be. *Regarding design:* • The website creates a professional image for the company, making it look reliable for commercial purposes. • It has a good layout. *Regarding navigation:* • Very nice, easy to navigate site. • Easy to browse. *Regarding speed:* • The download time is proficient for the website and pages load easily and quickly. • Loads quickly. • It's fast and efficient.
Negative	*Regarding function:* • There is no search capability or an FAQ section on various issues. • Searching for information was quite challenging. *Regarding design:* • The spinning buttons were a little annoying. • I find the changing of the images redundant. They do not support the purpose of the website.

Table 8.35 Participants' ideas regarding Web Site A (HTML version)

Polar	Ideas
Positive	*Regarding function:* • I think the links are all proper. • The content was very useful. • Pretty easy to follow, easy to understand. *Regarding design:* • The site looked nice. *Regarding navigation:* • There is adequate option to navigate between web pages.
Negative	*Regarding function:* • I found this site annoying, particularly in regards to finding out course information. • I found the search facility quite useless. *Regarding design:* • The links are not clear. They should be big and clear and catch visitors' attention immediately. • The "Contact" link is hidden way down the bottom of all pages. It took me ages to find it. *Regarding navigation:* • I found it hard to understand where I actually was. Especially in the course section. • Navigation bars are small and faint. • The main menu on the top should be more visible. *Regarding speed:* • The initial page took one minute to load.

Table 8.36 Participants' ideas regarding Web Site B (HTML version)

Polar	Ideas
Positive	*Regarding function:* • This site was easy to use. • The information was easy to find, and the process rewarding. • Allow spider searching. • I liked the content. *Regarding design:* • Nice colours and structure.
Negative	*Regarding design:* • There were a lot of graphics that made reading difficult. • The text is very tiring to read. It's too small. • The fonts are rather small. People with vision difficulties may find the words are too small to read. • The font, especially the main menu, should be larger. *Regarding navigation:* • Back button needed. • The navigation is not very effective. The hyperlinks down the left side were of no use as I had to keep going back to get to the home page to look up something new. • I didn't find a button that would go back/home which was annoying. *Regarding speed:* • Just took ages to load. Heavy graphics, not compressed enough.

Table 8.37 Participants' ideas regarding Web Site C (HTML version)

Polar	Ideas
Positive	*None*
Negative	*Regarding function:* • I thought the website was annoying and no where near flexible enough for international users. *Regarding design:* • I really disliked this website. The text was really small, making it very hard to read in some parts. • The font size is too small. • The fonts are too small and all are packed together. Eyes straining. • The fonts are too small to read. *Regarding navigation:* • Not a good site at all to navigate. *Regarding speed:* • Slow and occasionally doesn't load at all.

Table 8.38   Participants' ideas regarding Web Site D (HTML version)

Polar	Ideas
Positive	*Regarding function:* • Quite a nice and easy to use website. • The links in particular are very informative and well positioned. *Regarding design:* • The background has made the text unreadable. *Regarding navigation:* • The scrolling is annoying as I have to click on the arrow constantly to scroll up and down.
Negative	*Regarding design:* • This website is way too cluttered. *Regarding navigation:* • The scroll bar should have a bar that could tell the viewer where its ends. *Regarding speed:* • Very slow and clunky. Images sort of half load and give up. • Too many large graphics, too long to download. • It takes too long to load up onto my browser so it's not a web site that I would spend any time in.

Table 8.39   Participants' ideas regarding Web Site E (HTML version)

Polar	Ideas
Positive	*Regarding function:* • Search capabilities and results particularly useful. *Regarding navigation:* • The usability of this website is good. Easy to navigate
Negative	*Regarding navigation:* • The website itself was hard to navigate and was not easy to follow. • Navigating this web site was annoying, due to the fact that the navigation links are hidden on a dropdown list. • This site is sort of difficult to use. That the front page had little to no navigation options available to the user frustrated me. • It's very hard to understand as the menu is in a dropdown form.

Table 8.40 Participants' ideas regarding Web Site F (HTML version)

Polar	Ideas
Positive	*None*
Negative	*Regarding function:* • The links are a bit confusing. • No search available. • The links are messy. *Regarding design:* • The layout of some of the pages is a bit overwhelming and messy. *Regarding navigation:* • Annoying menu system, that is counter-intuitive in its operation. • Navigation was a little unintuitive. • Navigation a bit annoying.

The number of idea units in each category, for each Web site, was counted and tabulated, as shown in Table 8.41.

Table 8.41 Number of idea units after categorisation

Site	Flash Version										HTML Version									
	Positive					Negative					Positive					Negative				
	f	d	n	s	Σ	f	d	n	s	Σ	f	d	n	s	Σ	f	d	n	s	Σ
A	2	3	-	-	5	3	4	6	4	17	3	1	1	-	5	2	2	3	1	8
B	6	3	3	-	12	1	-	9	-	10	4	1	-	-	5	-	4	3	1	8
C	1	-	-	1	2	-	6	-	-	6	-	-	-	-	0	1	4	1	1	7
D	1	1	1	-	3	1	1	2	9	13	2	1	1	-	4	-	1	1	3	5
E	5	1	-	-	6	-	-	1	4	5	1	-	1	-	2	-	-	4	-	4
F	5	2	2	3	12	2	2	-	-	4	-	-	-	-	0	3	1	3	-	7
Σ	20	10	6	4	40	7	13	18	17	55	10	3	3	-	16	6	12	15	6	39

f = function, d = design, n = navigation, s = speed, Σ = total

This analysis can help explain the quantitative results, in terms of relative numbers of different sorts of comments, as well as reference to the details of the comments themselves. From Table 8.41, we can see that the number of negative opinions is higher than the number of positive opinions for both Flash and HTML Web sites, which is usual for many kinds of survey, as participants in general tend to comment more negatively than positively. In this case, the participants were asked to critically review the Web sites, which is probably why negative comments are in the majority. An interesting aspect in this analysis is that for Flash Web sites, the ratio between positive and negative comments is 40/55 (=0.73), while the same ratio for HTML Web sites is 16/39 (=0.41), i.e. the participants provided more positive comments for Flash Web sites than HTML Web sites. This supports the quantitative results found previously that Flash Web sites tend to display higher usability than HTML Web sites.

A more detailed analysis shows that for Flash Web sites, the positive comments (40) tended to be more about *function*, while the negative comments (55) were more about *navigation* and *speed*. This could be expected since Flash technology allows Web sites to incorporate multimedia contents (sounds, images, animations) seamlessly with other standard contents, and therefore they are able to provide more functionality and features to the users. One example is the Flash version of Web site A (Full Sail), which was praised by several participants in its functionality and design because it utilises the power of Flash to create a "virtual" guiding person, who introduces the Web site to the visitors and walks them through several parts of the site, as shown in Figure 8.17.

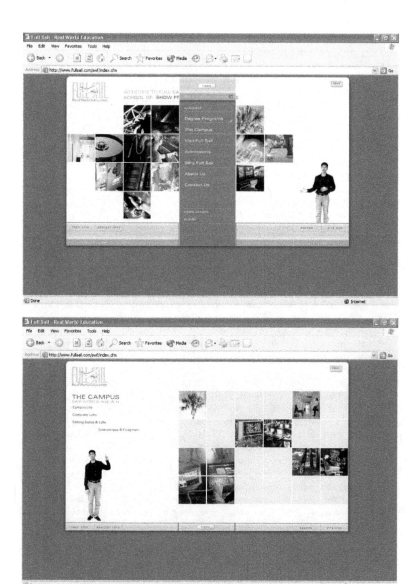

Figure 8.17 Screen capture of Web site A (Flash version) showing a virtual guiding person

Although audio-visual cues pervasive in Flash Web sites can be beneficial in accommodating or entertaining the users, sometimes they can also generate negative feelings towards the Web sites, as some users reported that moving images and/or sound effects were irritating to them. For instance, two participants expressed their feelings as follows:

"I found the taskbar to be very annoying as it pops up when you place your cursor over it. The sound effects became irritating." (Site A, Flash, Participant 1.12[1])

"I find the changing of the images redundant. They do not support the purpose of the website." (Site F, Flash, Participant 1.6)

However, some functions and features facilitated by Flash come with the cost of speed, as multimedia contents tend to be large in file size and require a considerable amount of time to download. This is reflected in several negative comments by the participants on downloading speed of Flash Web sites. For example, one participant commented that:

"It was an excruciating wait for the media to load." (Site D, Flash, Participant 1.20)

Although HTML Web sites could also suffer from slow downloading speed, it was to a lesser extent. Some Web sites which contain a considerable number of graphics and/or whose Web servers have limited capability of handling large amount of data transfer can suffer from slow downloading speed, regardless of whether Flash or HTML was used. For example, several participants commented negatively on download speed of Web site D, both Flash and HTML versions, while for some other Web sites there were only few or no negative comments at all regarding speed. The following comment was provided by a participant who visited the HTML version of the Web sites:

"It takes too long to load up onto my browser so it's not a web site that I would spend any time in." (Site D, HTML, Participant 1.23)

For the HTML Web sites, the positive comments (16) were mostly regarding *function* and the negative comments (39) were predominately concerning *design* and *navigation*. This could indicate that HTML Web sites could at least provide the same basic functionality that Flash Web sites could, but without extra multimedia-intensive contents. However, many users would still prefer Flash Web sites more because of their attractive designs that provide a positive first impression and an enjoyable experience, as one participant commented:

"The introductory animation/speech is great. It makes it both helpful and entertaining, which gives it an attractive first impression. I think this would work well with its target audience." (Site A, Flash, Participant 1.17)

For navigation, both Flash and HTML Web sites tend to suffer similarly from negative comments by the participants, and various users tend to have different opinions regarding this matter. Some users prefer navigation in Flash Web sites, while some users detest and feel resistant to it. This is because Flash Web sites mostly utilise non-standard navigation items (e.g. scrollbars, buttons, etc.), in contrast to HTML Web sites which mostly use standard navigation options provided

---

[1] Participant's demographic information can be found in Appendix 8A.

by the Web browser. One example is the Flash version of Web site B (Australians At War) which utilises a non-standard scrollbar for the timeline and a number of unlabelled buttons (as shown in Figure 8.18), which made some users feel uncomfortable. As an example, two participants provided the following statements:

"The movement and transition (the sliding effect) of the timeline made me feel uneasy and dizzy." (Site B, Flash, Participant 1.12)

"The yellow bullets were quite annoying because they were placed anywhere and they don't look like they lead to any links. There were no labels next to them nor were there any labels attached when the mouse is located over the top." (Site B, Flash, Participant 1.15)

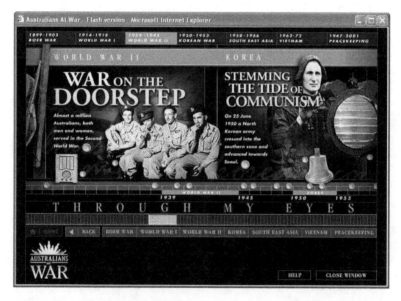

Figure 8.18 Screen capture of Web site B (Flash version) showing a non-standard scrollbar and unlabelled buttons

However, HTML Web sites can also face the same navigation challenge, even if they utilise standard navigation items, e.g. dropdown list. A few users commented that they found it difficult to navigate the HTML version of Web site E (Chronicle Books) because it utilised a dropdown list as the main menu, as shown in Figure 8.19. In some pages of the site, submenus were also presented one after another in dropdown form. One of the participants provided the following comment:

"Navigating this web site was annoying, due to the fact that the navigation links are hidden on a drop down list." (Site E, HTML, Participant 1.42)

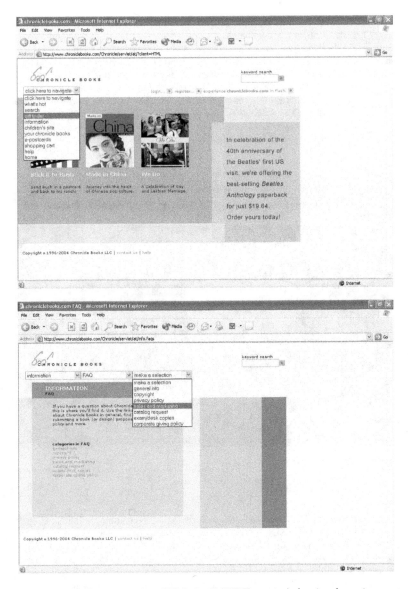

Figure 8.19 Screen capture of Web site E (HTML version) showing the main menu and submenus in dropdown form

One interesting point worth mentioning is that several users had conflicting opinions regarding the use of the standard "Back" button on a Web browser toolbar. Some users reported that they disliked Flash sites because the "Back" button could not be used to go back to the previous page (which is a common characteristic to all Flash Web sites). For instance, one participant pointed out that:

> "Pressing the 'back' button resets the homepage and doesn't go back to the content you chose." (Site B, Flash, Participant 1.12)

However, some users commented that they did not like some HTML Web sites that required them to use the "Back" button too often. Therefore, this suggests that the preference for this feature is more dependent on individual preference than on the version of Web sites.

In terms of the different types of Web sites (purpose), the contrast between positive versus negative comments was not clearly distinguishable, as there were only two Web sites per each category in this study. However, if a similar research study would be performed in the future, with a higher number of Web sites in each category, this analysis could also be useful as the number of positive and negative comments in each category could be significantly different and show some interesting patterns.

8.4 Usability of the Online Survey

After the participants had completed the online survey, they were asked to provide comments about the usability of the survey and procedures undertaken during the survey. Most of the participants were satisfied with how the survey was conducted and commented positively on the usability of the online survey. Many participants said that the survey was simple and easy to use, and that they could proceed through the survey without any difficulties. The layout of the survey was described as simple and clean, which in turn was considered professional and effective by most users.

However, there were several points mentioned by the participants that could be changed or improved if similar surveys are to be conducted in the future. These comments were grouped into two major categories, one regarding the implementation of the online survey, and the other regarding WUCET questions.

Comments regarding the implementation of the online survey:

- During the survey, each Web site to be evaluated was popped up in a new browser window, and when the user finished browsing the site, they had to switch to the other browser window containing the survey. Some users suggested that both the Web site and the survey should be presented in the same browser window, so they would not need to switch between browser windows too often. On the other hand, some participants said that they preferred to visit all Web sites first, and then complete the survey later, instead of interleaving Web sites into the survey.

- Some technical limitations of the online survey required the participants to complete the survey in one setting. However, some participants felt that it would be more beneficial to them if they could save their responses during the survey, leave the survey, and come back to continue at a later time/date. Some users also suggested that an automatic save feature (e.g. save after every five questions completed) be included in case of power failure or any other unexpected event/interruption.
- The navigation option of the survey was made so that the users could proceed to the next Web site only if they finished evaluating the current Web site. They could also go back to the evaluation questions of previous Web sites by clicking the "Previous" button once or multiple times, depending on how far back they would like to go. However, some users suggested that there should be more flexible navigation options, e.g. an option to jump to any specific part of the survey directly from any page of the survey.
- Several users commented that the survey was too long and consumed too much time to complete (one to two hours), as six Web sites had to be visited and the number of questions was approximately 20 per each Web site. Therefore, in the second experiment (eye tracking), the number of Web site was reduced to three Web sites and the average time used for each participant decreased to 30-45 minutes.

Comments regarding WUCET questions:

- In the survey, each WUCET question was given five answer choices: *strongly disagree, disagree, neutral, agree,* and *strongly agree.* However, some users suggested that one or more of the following choices also be included: *do not know, no opinion about this, do not understand the question, unable to judge, not applicable.*
- Some participants suggested that a grading system of 1 to 7 be used instead of five-point *strongly disagree* to *strongly agree,* as it could cater for a wider range of responses and also ease the burden of users having to "strongly" agree or disagree on something. On the other hand, some users felt that five-point scale was too much to choose from, as they found it difficult to distinguish between *(dis)agree* and *strongly (dis)agree.*
- For each Web site, WUCET questions were presented in random order. Some users commented that they preferred similar questions grouped together, and/or the questions should be presented in logical order, i.e. questions regarding download time or server status should be at the beginning of the survey as the users tend to be more aware of these factors when they first visit the Web site.
- Some participants commented that WUCET questions should have been all positively worded or negatively worded, or grouped into separate positive/negative groups, as they found the survey difficult and time-consuming to complete when positive and negative statements were randomly distributed. However, the reason WUCET statements were

presented that way was to get more accurate responses, because the respondents might have been less careful when completing the survey if all statements had been positively or negatively worded.

- In the survey, WUCET questions were presented as statements (e.g. This Web site is annoying.) and participants were asked to agree or disagree. However, some users said they would prefer the survey to use questions in direct interrogative form, to which they could respond yes or no (e.g. Do you find this Web site annoying?). Nonetheless, yes/no responses would have been less rigorous for data analysis if employed instead of five-point Likert scale.
- Several participants provided comments regarding some specific WUCET questions (statements), mostly because they found these questions difficult to respond to. The relevant questions and comments by the users are summarised in Table 8.42.

Table 8.42 Participants' comments on WUCET statements

WUCET Statement	Comment
The hyperlinks are all current.	It is impossible to check all links in the Web site, and the word "current" can be interpreted in many ways (e.g. link is working, or link is regarding current event).
Searching on this site yields good (and relevant) results.	Not applicable if the site does not have search facility.
The way searches are structured is not very useful.	Not applicable if the site does not have search facility.
You are able to find a help page, or help-related page quite easily.	Some users do not look for help so they could not answer.
Information presented at this site is complete.	It is difficult for the users to judge the completeness of the Web site, i.e. how complete is complete?
This web site is not accurate or truthful with the information presented.	Some users do not have background knowledge regarding contents of the Web site, so they do not know if they are accurate or not.
The content of this web site is useful for its intended purpose and audience.	The users have to guess the site's intended audience which can be difficult.
The server of this web-site is down or busy making browsing very slow or not effective.	Too technical terms (e.g. server down).
I have to use the latest version of the browser to get the most out of this site.	Some users could not answer this question as they did not try the Web site on any browser other than the one they are using, also they do not understand what is the most they should expect from the site.
This web site is not cluttered with unnecessary diagrams/graphics/etc.	Double negative statement, could be changed to "Are there too many diagrams/graphics?"
The layout of this web site lends itself to good planning of activities.	Ambiguous statement. Should it be the users or the designer who plan the activities?
I trust this web site enough to provide my Credit Card number, or personal information.	Not applicable to many Web sites where there are no purchases.
The layout of this web site does not adhere to standards/conventions.	Some users do not know what standards/conventions the Web site should follow.

8.5   Conclusion

This chapter discussed the analysis and results of the first experiment, which utilised a contingent heuristic approach via questionnaire. Both quantitative and qualitative methods were performed and significant findings were reported accordingly. Table 8.43 summarises the status of each hypothesis in regard to the tests performed.

Table 8.43   Summary of research hypotheses (Phase One)

Hypothesis	Status
H1: The Flash version of a Web site provides higher usability than the HTML version.	Supported
H2: Male users prefer the Flash version of a Web site (over the HTML version) to a greater extent than do female users.	Supported
H3: Users with shorter computer/Web experience prefer the Flash version of a Web site (over the HTML version) to a greater extent than do users with longer computer/Web experience.	Weakly supported
H4: Users with slower Internet connection speed see the difference in usability between the Flash and HTML versions of a Web site to a greater extent than do users with faster Internet connection speed.	Supported
H5: The category of a Web site (information, entertainment, e-commerce) affects the comparative usability of the Flash vs. HTML versions of the Web site.	Supported
H6: The version of a Web site visited (Flash or HTML) affects users' inclination and ability to perform tasks (use scenarios) within Web site, as reflected by the task completion score.	Weakly supported

In addition to the research hypotheses, the usability of the survey itself was also discussed with respect to commentary responses from the participants. The majority of the participants reported having a positive experience with the survey and several recommendations were provided for future improvements.

9

Results of the Phase Two Experiment (Eye Gaze Tracking)

9.1 Introduction

This chapter summarises the analyses and results of the second experiment, which utilised eye gaze tracking as a method for usability evaluation of Web sites. There were 39 participants involved in this experiment. Each participant visited the same three Web sites. However, 19 participants were asked to visit the Flash version of these Web sites, while the other 20 participants visited the HTML version. Since the participants had also been involved in the first experiment, each was allocated the opposite version of the Web sites to the version they had used in the first experiment. For details of the experimental procedure, see Chapter 7.

All participants' eye gaze patterns were recorded automatically with the remote eye gaze tracking equipment called *faceLAB* (version 3.2.1). Raw eye gaze data collected from the faceLAB system is in a binary form and contains various eye/head movement measurements. Therefore, it is necessary to extract only some data fields that are relevant to this study as the first step towards quantitative data analysis. The faceLAB eye tracking system records the user's eye gaze position at 60 Hz frequency, i.e. it captures the user's eye gaze every 1/60 of a second. Each time faceLAB captures eye gaze data, it writes that data to disk, together with a unique numeric identifier called *frame*. Frame number increases as more data is captured over time, and it is reset once the system is restarted (in this experiment, this was done every time a new participant came in, to prevent overflow in the frame number). During the experiment, a binary file with FLL extension (short for faceLAB Log) is created for each participant. It contains all data captured in a proprietary format (already compressed). The size of the data file depends on the duration of the experiment. The longer the experiment, the larger the file. On average, the size of a faceLAB log file is approximately one megabyte per minute recorded.

Seeing Machines, the provider of faceLAB, offers a software application named FaT (faceLAB Toolbox) which allows selected data (user-defined frame numbers and data fields) to be exported into an ASCII (text) file, which can be further analysed with other software applications, e.g. Microsoft Excel, SPSS. In this study, each log file (for each participant) was exported into three ASCII files, one for each Web site visited. The following data fields were selected for exporting because they were crucial to the analysis of Web site usability: frame number (for reference only), saccade, PERCLOS, and gaze-screen intersection. The saccade field contains a Boolean value (0 or 1), where 0 means there was no saccade detected during that frame, and 1 means there was a saccade. PERCLOS is a fatigue measure endorsed by the National Highway Traffic Safety Administration (U.S. Department of Transportation), which is the percentage of the intervals with closed eyes in a fixed time window (disregarding regular blinks). PERCLOS values range between 0 and 1. For example, if a user has 5 eye closures of 3 seconds each (for a total of 15 seconds) within a 60-second period, his/her PERCLOS value is 0.25 (=15/60). The gaze-screen intersection field contains a Boolean value, where 0 means that the user's eye gaze did not intersect with the computer screen, while 1 means the opposite. Therefore, it is particularly useful for checking whether the user is looking at the screen or away from it.

Once the required data was extracted, it was imported into Microsoft Excel for further analysis. First, the gaze-screen intersection field was used to filter out any frame that the user's eye gaze fell out of the screen area (gaze-screen intersection = 0), as shown in Figure 9.1 (removed frames in reverted colours). For the sake of simplicity, only 30 frames are shown in this example.

Frame	Saccade	PERCLOS	Gaze-Screen Intersection
37617	0	0.006272	1
37618	0	0.006272	1
37619	1	0.006272	1
37620	1	0.006272	0
37621	1	0.006272	0
37622	1	0.006272	0
37623	1	0.006272	1
37624	0	0.006266	1
37625	0	0.006266	1
37626	0	0.006266	1
37627	0	0.006266	1
37628	0	0.006266	1
37629	1	0.006265	1
37630	1	0.006265	0
37631	0	0.006265	0
37632	0	0.006265	0
37633	0	0.006265	1
37634	0	0.006265	1
37635	0	0.006265	1
37636	1	0.006265	1
37637	1	0.006268	1
37638	0	0.006268	1
37639	0	0.006268	1
37640	0	0.006268	1
37641	0	0.006268	1
37642	0	0.006268	1
37643	0	0.006268	1
37644	0	0.006268	1
37645	1	0.006269	1
37646	0	0.006269	1

Frame	Saccade	PERCLOS	Gaze-Screen Intersection
37617	0	0.006272	1
37618	0	0.006272	1
37619	1	0.006272	1
37623	1	0.006272	1
37624	0	0.006266	1
37625	0	0.006266	1
37626	0	0.006266	1
37627	0	0.006266	1
37628	0	0.006266	1
37629	1	0.006265	1
37633	0	0.006265	1
37634	0	0.006265	1
37635	0	0.006265	1
37636	1	0.006265	1
37637	1	0.006268	1
37638	0	0.006268	1
37639	0	0.006268	1
37640	0	0.006268	1
37641	0	0.006268	1
37642	0	0.006268	1
37643	0	0.006268	1
37644	0	0.006268	1
37645	1	0.006269	1
37646	0	0.006269	1

Figure 9.1 Example of eye tracking data showing the removal of the frames in which the user was not looking inside the screen area

After the unwanted frames were removed, fixations were extracted by using the information from the saccade field. This method was chosen because fixation information was not available directly from the faceLAB system. However, Seeing Machines, the provider of faceLAB, suggested that at any time when there was no saccade (saccade = 0), there had to be fixation. Therefore, the number of consecutive frames with no saccade was counted as one fixation and the duration of each fixation (in seconds) was calculated by dividing the number of frames in the fixation by 60 (as the gaze data was recorded at the rate of 60 frames per second). Fixation before the first saccade or after the last saccade was omitted because its length could not be determined (incomplete fixation). This makes the first real fixation happen after the first saccade and the last real fixation happen before the last saccade. For the same reason, any incomplete fixation occurred immediately before the user looking out of the screen or immediately after the user looking back into the screen was also removed. The fixation extraction process is shown in Figure 9.2. Gray-highlighted rows reflect complete fixations used for further analyses, while incomplete fixations (omitted from the analyses) are shown in reverted colours. A Visual Basic macro was written to help automate the extraction process within Excel (source code is provided in Appendix 9A).

Frame	Saccade	PERCLOS	Gaze-Screen Intersection
37617	0	0.006272	1
37618	0	0.006272	1
37619	1	0.006272	1
37623	1	0.006272	1
37624	0	0.006266	1
37625	0	0.006266	1
37626	0	0.006266	1
37627	0	0.006266	1
37628	0	0.006266	1
37629	1	0.006265	1
37633	0	0.006265	1
37634	0	0.006265	1
37635	0	0.006265	1
37636	1	0.006265	1
37637	1	0.006268	1
37638	0	0.006268	1
37639	0	0.006268	1
37640	0	0.006268	1
37641	0	0.006268	1
37642	0	0.006268	1
37643	0	0.006268	1
37644	0	0.006268	1
37645	1	0.006269	1
37646	0	0.006269	1

Frame	Number of Frames	Fixation Duration (sec)
37624-37628	5	0.0833
37638-37644	7	0.1167

Figure 9.2 Example of eye tracking data showing the extraction of fixation data

For the usability evaluation of a computer user interface, including Web sites, several eye gaze measures can be used, as discussed in Chapter 5. However, only the following measures were selected for this study because they were effective in measuring Web site usability and supported by the faceLAB system:

1. **Average fixation duration.** This is the average duration of all fixations over the period of viewing the Web site. Average fixation duration is the most frequently used measure for usability evaluation, as it is accepted that more complex information/representation usually requires a higher level of processing and therefore leads to longer fixation duration time. This is emphasised by Goldberg and Kotval (1999)

who claim that representations which require long fixations are not as meaningful to the user as those with shorter fixation durations.

2. **Cumulative fixation time per second.** Cumulative fixation time is the sum of duration of all fixations over the period of viewing the Web site. Cowen, Ball, and Delin (2002) have suggested that cumulative fixation time (they call it *total fixation duration*) is a global measure of the total amount of processing performed on each page (or in this study, each Web site), rather than just the mean amount of processing on each part of a page (or a Web site). However, since different users spend different amounts of time viewing the same Web site, this cumulative fixation time is divided by the total amount of time viewing the Web site, so that the cumulative fixation time of each person is comparable to others. Cumulative fixation time per second can also be calculated by summing the total number of fixation frames and dividing it with the total number of all frames; this method was implemented in the analysis of this experiment.

3. **Number of fixations per second.** The number of fixations is the total number of individual fixations over the period of viewing the Web site. Tzanidou (2003) suggests that an increase in the number of fixations indicates the difficulty in extracting information or the frustration of the interaction with the user interface. However, the number of fixations could also indicate the amount of interest in a specific area of the screen. For the same reason as the previous measure, the total number of fixations is divided by the time used for viewing the Web site, to provide the number of fixations per second.

4. **Average PERCLOS.** This is the average PERCLOS value over the period of viewing the Web site. PERCLOS is an effective indicator of fatigue (or alertness), as it is the percentage of eyelid closure over the pupil over time and reflects slow eyelid closures (droops) rather than blinks (Federal Highway Administration, 1998). The higher the value, the greater tiredness indicated. PERCLOS measurement is often used in detecting a driver's alertness while driving a motor vehicle. However, it is hypothesised that PERCLOS could also be used in user interface evaluation as well, because the effectiveness of a user interface should have a negative relationship with the user's boredom (lack of engagement), whose effect is very similar to that of the user's fatigue.

9.2 Quantitative Analysis

After the measurement data was calculated for each participant, quantitative analysis was performed by considering Web site version (Flash/HTML), category (information/entertainment/e-commerce), and users' gender as independent variables, while eye gaze tracking measures, as discussed in the previous section, were regarded as dependent variables. The following research questions and hypotheses were tested according to the quantitative eye gaze data collected from the experiment:

Q7: Are users' eye gaze measures affected by Web site version viewed (Flash or HTML)?

H7: Users' eye gaze measures can be affected by Web site version viewed (Flash or HTML).

Q8: Are users' eye gaze measures affected by category of Web site version viewed (information, entertainment, or e-commerce)?

H8: Users' eye gaze measures can be affected by category of Web site version viewed (information, entertainment, or e-commerce).

Q9: Are users' eye gaze measures determined by gender?

H9: Users' eye gaze measures can be determined by gender.

Table 9.1 depicts descriptive statistics of eye gaze measurements considered in this study, while Figures 9.3-9.6 show corresponding distribution histograms.

Table 9.1   Descriptive statistics of eye gaze variables

Variable	Number of Cases	Minimum	Maximum	Mean	Std. Deviation
Average Fixation Duration	117	.629	4.787	1.834	.771
Cumulative Fixation Time per Second	117	.790	.985	.941	.035
Number of Fixations per Second	117	.204	1.336	.601	.238
Average PERCLOS	117	.000	.140	.022	.032

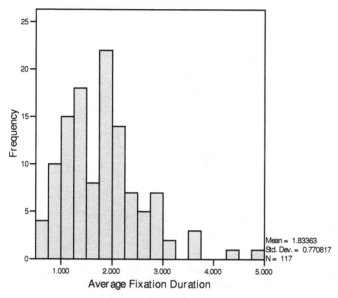

Figure 9.3   Histogram showing the distribution of average fixation duration

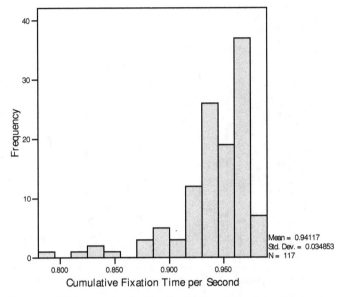

Figure 9.4 Histogram showing the distribution of cumulative fixation time per second

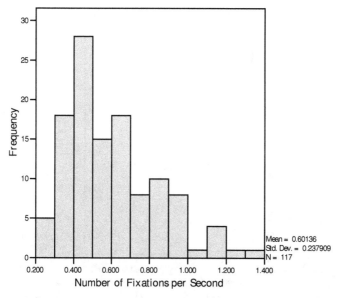

Figure 9.5 Histogram showing the distribution of number of fixations per second

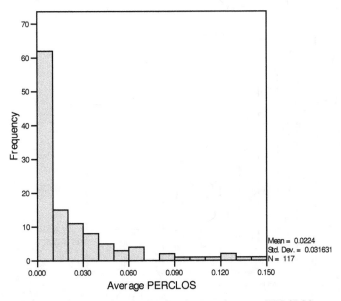

Figure 9.6   Histogram showing the distribution of average PERCLOS

In order to test the hypotheses, the combined situation of all Web sites was considered because the number of cases in this experiment was not high enough to conduct the tests for each Web site individually.

For the testing of hypothesis H7, all cases were separated in to two groups, according to the Web site version visited. Table 9.2 displays descriptive statistics of the dependent variables after this grouping.

Table 9.2   Descriptive statistics of eye gaze variables (grouped by site version)

Variable	Version	Number of Cases	Mean	Std. Deviation	Mean Difference (Flash-HTML)
Average Fixation Duration	Flash	57	1.891	.848	.111
	HTML	60	1.780	.693	
Cumulative Fixation Time per Second	Flash	57	.937	.044	-.008
	HTML	60	.945	.023	
Number of Fixations per Second	Flash	57	.602	.273	.001
	HTML	60	.601	.201	
Average PERCLOS	Flash	57	.024	.036	.004
	HTML	60	.021	.027	

From Table 9.2, it can be inferred that the average fixation duration is longer in the Flash version than in the HTML version. On the other hand, cumulative fixation time per second is longer in the HTML version. For the other two measures, the standard deviations are so high that they outweigh the differences in means. This can be clarified by performing independent t-tests (two-tailed), as shown in Table 9.3.

Table 9.3   Results from independent t-tests comparing eye gaze variables by site version (Flash-HTML)

Variable	Equal Variances	t	df	Sig. (2-tailed)	Mean Difference	Std. Error Difference
Average Fixation Duration	assumed	.777	115	.439	.111	.143
	not assumed	.773	108.250	.441	.111	.144
Cumulative Fixation Time per Second	assumed	-1.297	115	.197	-.008	.006
	not assumed	-1.279	84.761	.205	-.008	.007
Number of Fixations per Second	assumed	.030	115	.976	.001	.044
	not assumed	.030	102.592	.976	.001	.045
Average PERCLOS	assumed	.610	115	.543	.004	.006
	not assumed	.605	104.329	.546	.004	.006

Table 9.3 suggests that there is no significant difference in any eye gaze measure between Flash and HTML Web sites. This could be caused by the high standard deviations within each group and the low number of participants. Therefore, hypothesis H7 is not supported by the empirical evidence of this study.

In order to test hypothesis H8, cases were grouped according to the Web site visited, as there were three Web sites, each of which falls in a different category. In this case, paired-sample t-tests were performed because each participant had visited all three Web sites. Comparisons between the information site and the entertainment site (A-B), between the entertainment site and the e-commerce site (B-C), and between the information site and the e-commerce site (A-C) were made, as shown in Tables 9.4, 9.5, and 9.6, respectively.

Table 9.4   Results from paired t-tests comparing eye gaze variables between information and entertainment Web sites (A-B)

Variable	Mean of Difference	Std. Deviation	Std. Error Mean	t	df	Sig. (2-tailed)
Average Fixation Duration	.019	.486	.078	.244	38	.808
Cumulative Fixation Time per Second	-.007	.028	.004	-1.661	38	.105
Number of Fixations per Second	.010	.176	.028	.367	38	.716
Average PERCLOS	-.004	.021	.003	-1.234	38	.225

Table 9.5   Results from paired t-tests comparing eye gaze variables between entertainment and e-commerce Web sites (B-C)

Variable	Mean of Difference	Std. Deviation	Std. Error Mean	t	df	Sig. (2-tailed)
Average Fixation Duration	.240	.505	.081	2.967	38	.005***
Cumulative Fixation Time per Second	.013	.032	.005	2.500	38	.017**
Number of Fixations per Second	-.061	.142	.023	-2.661	38	.011**
Average PERCLOS	-.005	.020	.003	-1.495	38	.143

** = significant at .05 level, *** = significant at .01 level

Table 9.6   Results from paired t-tests comparing eye gaze variables between information and e-commerce Web sites (A-C)

Variable	Mean of Difference	Std. Deviation	Std. Error Mean	t	df	Sig. (2-tailed)
Average Fixation Duration	.259	.682	.109	2.368	38	.023**
Cumulative Fixation Time per Second	.005	.037	.006	.912	38	.367
Number of Fixations per Second	-.050	.213	.034	-1.471	38	.150
Average PERCLOS	-.009	.024	.004	-2.303	38	.027**

** = significant at .05 level

As shown in Table 9.4, no significant difference was found in the eye gaze variables between information and entertainment Web sites. However, there are significant differences in average fixation duration between entertainment and e-commerce Web sites, and also between information and e-commerce Web sites, i.e. participant's fixation duration was shorter in the e-commerce Web site than the other two Web sites. This could be because the e-commerce Web site is more organised, so that the user does not need to fixate on specific areas of the site for so long to understand what they represent. The significant difference in cumulative fixation time between entertainment and e-commerce Web sites can also be interpreted the same way, as cumulative fixation time also indicates the amount of processing required to understand the representations. The lower number of fixations in the entertainment Web site (compared to the e-commerce Web site) could be resulting from longer fixation durations, because when fixations are counted during a specific period of time, longer fixations usually generate a smaller counted number. In addition, the e-commerce Web site incurred a significantly higher average PERCLOS value than the information Web site. This could indicate that the e-commerce Web site is less interesting to these users than the information Web site, and therefore engages the user less strongly.

According to these significant differences found in some eye gaze measures across the Web sites, it could be concluded that hypothesis H8 is weakly supported. Although the order of viewing the Web sites was the same for all participants (Web site A, then B, then C), the possible effects of Web site order on eye gaze behaviours were found to be minimal, because there were only three Web sites used in the experiment and no significant difference in eye gaze variables was found between the first two Web sites. In addition, one Web site selected for each category may seem to be a small representative of Web sites in that category; however, the selection was carefully made based on users' feedback from the first experiment, so that the chosen Web sites could well represent their category.

Hypothesis H9 was tested in the same manner as hypothesis H7, except that all cases were separated into gender groups instead of Flash/HTML groups. Table 9.7 shows the descriptive statistics of eye gaze variables for this hypothesis and Table 9.8 shows corresponding t-test results.

Table 9.7 Descriptive statistics of eye gaze variables (grouped by gender)

Variable	Gender	Number of Cases	Mean	Std. Deviation	Mean Difference (Female-Male)
Average Fixation Duration	Female	45	1.701	.796	-.215
	Male	72	1.916	.749	
Cumulative Fixation Time per Second	Female	45	.937	.032	-.007
	Male	72	.944	.036	
Number of Fixations per Second	Female	45	.651	.250	.081
	Male	72	.570	.226	
Average PERCLOS	Female	45	.014	.017	-.014
	Male	72	.028	.037	

Table 9.8 Results from independent t-tests comparing eye gaze variables by gender (Female-Male)

Variable	Equal Variances	t	df	Sig. (2-tailed)	Mean Difference	Std. Error Difference
Average Fixation Duration	assumed	-1.474	115	.143	-.215	.146
	not assumed	-1.453	89.249	.150	-.215	.148
Cumulative Fixation Time per Second	assumed	-1.114	115	.267	-.007	.007
	not assumed	-1.143	101.247	.256	-.007	.006
Number of Fixations per Second	assumed	1.809	115	.073*	.081	.045
	not assumed	1.767	86.346	.081*	.081	.046
Average PERCLOS	assumed	-2.343	115	.021**	-.014	.006
	not assumed	-2.740	106.009	.007***	-.014	.005

* = significant at .10 level, ** = significant at .05 level, *** = significant at .01 level

Table 9.8 suggests that female users tend to have a higher number of fixations than males (at .10 significant level), within the same period of time. This could result from shorter average fixation durations. However, the difference in average fixation duration between male and female users cannot be significantly inferred from the results. Regarding the PERCLOS measure, males tend to have higher PERCLOS values than females, which indicates that male users can be less engaged than females when browsing the Web sites.

From the significant differences in the number of fixations and PERCLOS between males and females, it can be seen that hypothesis H9 is weakly supported.

9.3 Preference for Web Site Versions (Flash or HTML)

When the eye gaze tracking experiment was completed, each participant was asked to rate his/her personal preference for the Flash or HTML version of the three Web sites. Each response was coded into a numerical value (preference score) as follows:

- Flash version is a lot better = 5
- Flash version is a little bit better = 4
- Both versions are equally good = 3
- HTML version is a little bit better = 2
- HTML version is a lot better = 1

Then the average of the preference scores was computed for each Web site. The information Web site (Full Sail) has an average of 3.49. The entertainment Web site (Madonna) has an average of 3.64. The e-commerce Web site (Chronicle Books) has an average of 3.23. Thus, the participants overall prefer the Flash version to the HTML version of all Web sites. However, the preference for Flash version is more dominant in the entertainment Web site than the other two Web sites. This could imply that entertainment Web sites are more suitable to be implemented in Flash, because the users expect to see intensive audio-visual contents in these Web sites, which could be catered for better by Flash than by standard HTML format. For information Web sites, preference for Flash version over HTML version is also evident albeit not as strong as entertainment Web sites. Regarding e-commerce Web sites, the Flash version could also make the shopping experience more enjoyable for users, e.g. the presentation of merchandise is usually more appealing in Flash Web sites than in HTML Web sites. However, the difference between the two versions may be so subtle that many users rated both of them equally.

In addition, further categorisation was made so that the participants were separated into two gender groups. Table 9.9 shows the average preference score for each Web site after this grouping.

Table 9.9   Average preference score for each Web site, categorised by gender

Group	Number of Participants	Average Preference Score		
		Information Site (Full Sail)	Entertainment Site (Madonna)	E-Commerce Site (Chronicle Books)
Female	15	3.33	3.60	3.47
Male	24	3.58	3.67	3.08
Total	39	3.49	3.64	3.23

From Table 9.9, it can be seen that males and females have almost equal preference for the Flash version of the entertainment Web site, while male participants prefer the Flash version of the information Web site to a greater extent than female participants (although not by much). For the e-commerce Web site, females tend to prefer the Flash version while males prefer both versions equally. This could be because females are generally more sensitive when doing shopping than males, and therefore are more likely to find the benefits of Flash over HTML in e-commerce Web sites. However, because of the small number of participants and the fact that users' preference was transformed from categorical to numerical value, the difference in preference score between both gender groups could not be asserted quantitatively by corresponding t-tests, as shown in Table 9.10.

Table 9.10   Results from independent t-tests comparing preference score for each Web site between female and male participants

Web Site	Equal Variances	t	df	Sig. (2-tailed)	Mean Difference	Std. Error Difference
A (Full Sail)	assumed	-.591	37	.558	-.250	.423
	not assumed	-.580	28.158	.566	-.250	.431
B (Madonna)	assumed	-.173	37	.864	-.067	.386
	not assumed	-.172	29.553	.865	-.067	.387
C (Chronicle Books)	assumed	1.049	37	.301	.383	.365
	not assumed	1.149	36.772	.258	.383	.334

In addition to the numerical analysis, it is also useful to analyse the responses categorically. Therefore the number of responses for each Web site, categorised by preference and gender category, was tallied and summarised in Table 9.11.

Table 9.11 Number of responses, categorised by preference and gender

Preference	Female				Male				Combined			
	Site A	Site B	Site C	All Sites	Site A	Site B	Site C	All Sites	Site A	Site B	Site C	All Sites
Flash version is a lot better (a)	3	4	2	9 (20%)	7	7	2	16 (22%)	10 (26%)	11 (28%)	4 (10%)	25 (21%)
Flash version is a little bit better (b)	5	5	4	14 (31%)	7	7	9	23 (32%)	12 (31%)	12 (31%)	13 (33%)	37 (32%)
Both versions are equally good (c)	3	2	8	13 (29%)	4	6	6	16 (22%)	7 (18%)	8 (21%)	14 (36%)	29 (25%)
HTML version is a little bit better (d)	2	4	1	7 (16%)	5	3	3	11 (15%)	7 (18%)	7 (18%)	4 (10%)	18 (15%)
HTML version is a lot better (e)	2	0	0	2 (4%)	1	1	4	6 (8%)	3 (8%)	1 (3%)	4 (10%)	8 (7%)
Flash version is better (a+b)	8	9	6	23 (51%)	14	14	11	39 (54%)	22 (56%)	23 (59%)	17 (44%)	62 (53%)
HTML version is better (d+e)	4	4	1	9 (20%)	6	4	7	17 (24%)	10 (26%)	8 (21%)	8 (21%)	26 (22%)
Total	15	15	15	45	24	24	24	72	39	39	39	117

From Table 9.11, it can be inferred that, overall, the majority of the participants prefer the Flash version of the Web sites more than the HTML version (53% versus 22%), and within the 53% who prefer Flash, 40% (25 out of 62) prefer it to a greater extent than the rest. For each individual Web site, A (information site), B (entertainment site), and C (e-commerce site), the majority of the participants also prefer the Flash version to the HTML version at 56%, 59%, and 44%, respectively. This supports the result in the first experiment that entertainment Web sites tend to be more preferred in Flash version than any other type of Web sites. However, the situation between the information and e-commerce Web sites is not conformable to the result of the first experiment. In the first experiment, it was found that e-commerce Web sites produced significant difference in usability between Flash and HTML versions, while information Web sites did not show the same significance. This non-conformity could result from the fact that the number of Web sites was reduced to half in the second experiment, and the information Web site selected for the second experiment (Full Sail) was very well applauded by the users in its usability of the Flash version, especially when compared to the other information Web site that was omitted from the second experiment, to the extent that the effect of this Web site is stronger than that of the e-commerce Web site.

Regarding different gender groups, both male and female participants seem to prefer the Flash version of the Web sites more than the HTML version alike (54% vs. 24%, and 51% vs. 20%, respectively). However, there are more females who considered both versions equally good than males (29% vs. 22%). This can be seen as partial support for the result from the first experiment, where females saw less significant difference between the usability of Flash and HTML Web sites and therefore tend to rate both versions equally.

In addition to the five-point rating scale, the participants were also asked to provide comments on each Web site to support their preference selection. Tables 9.12-9.14 present these commentary responses according to the participants' preference, categorised by gender.

Table 9.12 Commentary responses for Full Sail (information) Web site

Preference	Comments from Female Users	Comments from Male Users
Flash version is a lot better	• It is more interesting and the set up is more professional in look and features. I also liked the introduction with the little man. • I liked this website in Flash because it was more interesting.	• It provides an easy flowing interface that doesn't have to change screens every click. It also provides a more 'eye candy' effect and this attracts many different users. • I find that Flash is better for entertainment value. The video at the start is really good. • I like the animated style of this page. • The HTML design is poor. • Some of the links [on the HTML version] are not very clear to see.
Flash version is a little bit better	• It seemed to be a little more entertaining instead of just plain text with an accompanying image shown in the HTML version. • I liked the Flash version a little bit better because it fits the site and it is not too annoying. • More animation which guides your attention.	• I felt that the Flash version of the site worked better, as it better suited the subject matter of Full Sail. • Harder to find the FAQ section than the HTML version. Site looks a lot nicer and more cutting edge. • The Flash version is certainly a lot more helpful (the little video guy is a nice touch) but on first use, the menu is a little difficult to understand. • The little guy that came on the screen was a nice touch. It personalises it and makes the viewer more relaxed/welcomed. • Due to the nature of Full Sail, a multimedia representation of the campus is more appropriate. It's more attractive and I found the HTML version to be exceedingly static.

Preference	Comments from Female Users	Comments from Male Users
Both versions are equally good	• This is because there isn't much difference between the both versions, in terms of interactivity and structure. • Flash version is definitely more interesting but there wasn't a button to go back to the previous screen. And sometimes the response is slow compared to HTML page. • Flash looks better but HTML is easier to navigate.	• Flash was great, HTML was just as good (for HTML anyway). • Both versions have its one odd and good reason. It's much quicker to locate information in the HTML format, but much interesting for surfing information in the Flash version. • I don't really have a preference between Flash or HTML version for this site. Equally the same. • The information I want was equally present in both versions.
HTML version is a little bit better	• The HTML version made me more comfortable to browse the site because things wouldn't be popping and moving on the screen all the time. I felt like I had more time to explore the site and find the information I was after. • Flash download time took too long.	• Quicker. • The HTML did not take time to download as it was quite simple and straight to the point. In other words, you are sure that your viewers won't get caught up in the design and would be able to accomplish their tasks in no potential design problems. • I found the animations in the Flash version to be a little irritating. Same with the fancy animations and interface. The HTML version was a lot more straightforward and easy to navigate through. • Looking for information about school, the structure in HTML gives me more confident in making decision.
HTML version is a lot better	• HTML version is easier to understand. • Flash version was too confusing to use. Not a conventional way to organise an interface.	• Much preferred the HTML version, like my status bar [was enabled] for one thing.

Table 9.13 Commentary responses for Madonna (entertainment) Web site

Preference	Comments from Female Users	Comments from Male Users
Flash version is a lot better	• For this web site, the Flash version was a lot more attractive to me. It made the site more dynamic, and I think it fits with Madonna's media image. Modern, vibrant, and constantly on the move. • Moving graphics is a lot better with the Flash site. • Sound and animation guide your attention and it is more interesting.	• The music industry is all about looking pretty. So the Flash website fits in with the overall presentation of Madonna. • I like the Flash version because the music plays well. • The [HTML] page seemed cluttered and harder to navigate. • Different kinds of interaction with Flash version. More interactive. • Really hated the HTML version, not a huge fan of the Flash version, but it is a marked improvement.
Flash version is a little bit better	• The structure in Flash version is better than HTML version. And music is added in the Flash version. • I liked this website better than the HTML site but it was a little harder to find the requested info and I was distracted by the sound file. Has a really nice look and the menu options quite stylish. • Once again it was interesting. However it can be a bit distracting. But it is better than HTML. • [Regarding both versions,] no indication of how far down the page you are when scrolling through the site. Hard to know when you're at the end of the document.	• It's a little bit better, because it had music, and very interactive. • Not too different to the HTML version. The HTML version was a good replication of the Flash edition. Better use of images and sound on the Flash version. • The Flash version in this case suits the theme of a music artist's website and therefore is more suitable to implement. The Flash website does not take too long to download and is equal to the HTML version in terms of download time. • The background music is appropriate to a musician's homepage. • The Flash seems to give the artiste more depth.
Both versions are equally good	• There seemed to be little difference between the two versions except in appearance. • Both are interactive.	• These are quite similar, but I can do without the music [on the Flash version]. • I didn't notice any real difference (i.e. loading times of sites). • Surprisingly the difference visually is hardly noticeable. • There wasn't a great deal of difference between the two versions as far as I could see. • The background behind the text made it quite hard to read. Both sites seem to be quite similar except the Flash version has sound and animation.

Preference	Comments from Female Users	Comments from Male Users
HTML version is a little bit better	• [Regarding the Flash version,] the navigation bar at the bottom is not very useful as user has to move the cursor to the links, wait for 3 seconds then only the link appear. A little slow. And I couldn't get back to the previous screen because no 'Back' button. • HTML loads quicker but both are relatively easy to navigate. • I liked the HTML version better because the Flash version is just too annoying, too many Flashing images all the time. • Flash download time was too long.	• Faster to load, but browsing is the same speed. • The Flash version takes too long time to load.
HTML version is a lot better	*None*	• The Flash version was an excruciating wait for loading times.

Table 9.14 Commentary responses for Chronicle Books (e-commerce) Web site

Preference	Comments from Female Users	Comments from Male Users
Flash version is a lot better	• The HTML version seemed to run sluggishly. The feedback seemed faster in the Flash version • Just with the design of the menus, you don't need to click on it and then click on a category - you can see what the categories are in the drop down menu.	• I think I just prefer Flash websites.
Flash version is a little bit better	• I liked both websites although I think that the Flash is more interesting and stylistic. HTML is obviously a lot easier to use. • In one way I like the HTML version because it does not take that long time to visit the different pages and it fits with the purpose of the site. However, the Flash version makes the layout look better and it is easier to get an overview of the different pages. • I enjoyed the Flash and the download time was not as bad as other Flash sites.	• These are both a bit slow, but you get more a sense of progression and that something is happening in the Flash version. • Although the Flash is better interactive wise, the HTML serves as a better ground for categorical situations. • Easier to find books in certain categories. • Flash version is a little better, however that site seemed a bit slow when updating your choices. • I found the HTML version of this page almost impossible to navigate. It is almost as if HTML was an afterthought and no real money or time was spent developing it to the same level as the Flash version. • The Flash site had a better feel to it and the menu design was a lot easier to understand and navigate. • I liked the Flash version better but the loading time for the Flash movies were sometimes a little too long. But over all it was an ok site.

Preference	Comments from Female Users	Comments from Male Users
Both versions are equally good	• I don't think it makes much of a difference being Flash or HTML for this site. Maybe it's the content. If you're looking for a book, all you need is readily available on both versions, and the information is pretty easy to find. Perhaps the fact that I'd have a specific book in mind make my actions on this web site more predictable, when compared to the leisure browsing of Madonna's site, where I could be just looking for some entertainment. • Just slow, slow in looking up the database, fonts are too small. The graphics are distractive. • Both were easy to navigate and looked quite similar. • Little unsure how to get to the different pages on the site. I think the mouse over technique [on the Flash version] could be a little confusing. • I like both because they are easy to understand. • Both structured fairly well, both are easy to use. • I think they are the same.	• Both had a really good and similar design, and both work well and are easy to understand. • It looks nice, but I think it's faster on the HTML page. • The site is comprehensive in both its incarnations.
HTML version is a little bit better	• In Flash site, I got to wait for the next page to be loaded which I thought is quite unusual for site using Flash. HTML is better, in the sense that everything is kept very simple and easy to understand.	• The theme of the website is to sell books online and therefore the website should be kept simple and in this case I would say that the HTML version is more suitable and better as it generally allows viewers to complete their tasks such as buying books in a simple and efficient way. The Flash version is also good but it takes sometime to download and the design is a bit too much at times. Therefore the HTML version is recommendable in this case and allows viewers to enjoy their browsing experience. • The HTML version does not need to load anything from the server, saves a lot of time. • If I want to make a serious purchase and maybe more after that, HTML seems to provide me with more confident, HTML seems more consistent and consistency breeds reliability.

Preference	Comments from Female Users	Comments from Male Users
HTML version is a lot better	*None*	• Because of the download time it takes to bring out the information on the screen, [the Flash version] is really bad. I would prefer HTML version over Flash, any time. • Flash version is too slow when loading. • Less errors in HTML. • I didn't like the Flash version.

The comments from the participants seem to be compatible with those of the first experiment, i.e. the Flash version of the Web sites was much preferred mostly because of its attractive and interactive design, which utilises sound and animation to make the user more engaged and entertained while browsing the Web. For instance, one participant commented concisely that:

> "Sound and animation guide your attention and it is more interesting [than the HTML version]." (Site B, Participant 2.37)

One of the advantages of Flash technology discovered from the participants' comments is that Flash allows individual contents of the Web site to be updated independently without the need to load the whole page like in HTML Web sites, which can make the browsing experience of the user more flowing (less interruption), as one participant pointed out that:

> "[The Flash version] provides an easy flowing interface that doesn't have to change screens every click. It also provides a more 'eye candy' effect and this attracts many different users." (Site A, Participant 2.13)

A research study by Stanford-Poynter (2000) also reported that for HTML Web sites, users tend to interlace multiple Web sites while browsing (switch back and forth between them), which may be because they feel that every HTML page is separated from another (physically and logically) and this situation should not be present in Flash Web sites. However, this could only be confirmed by further research.

On the negative side of Flash usability, similar to the first experiment, navigation and speed issues are still dominantly present. Navigation options in Flash Web sites tend to be difficult to understand (especially when first visited) and/or utilise unnecessary animated effects. For example, two users provided the following comments:

> "The Flash version is certainly a lot more helpful but on first use, the menu is a little difficult to understand." (Site A, Participant 2.10)

> "[Regarding the Flash version,] the navigation bar at the bottom is not very useful as user has to move the cursor to the links, wait for 3 seconds then only the link appear." (Site B, Participant 2.8)

Therefore, it could be inferred that although users prefer the animation and sound in Flash Web sites, navigation should be kept simple and consistent, as the users usually look for interactivity in the contents, not in the navigation items.

Regarding HTML Web sites, several users commented negatively on the design (look and feel) because they thought it was too static or too plain to see. For example, two of the participants pointed out that:

"Due to the nature of Full Sail, a multimedia representation of the campus is more appropriate. It's more attractive and I found the HTML version to be exceedingly static." (Site A, Participant 2.21)

"[The Flash version] seemed to be a little more entertaining instead of just plain text with an accompanying image shown in the HTML version." (Site A, Participant 2.26)

On the other hand, the download speed of HTML Web sites was much appreciated as it is common for Flash Web sites to be larger in size and therefore require longer time to download than HTML Web sites. However, from another point of view, download speed could be considered an external variable, as it is not inherent in the Flash technology but dependent mostly on Internet connection. Furthermore, in the near future when more users utilise high-speed Internet connection, the difference in the download speed of Flash versus HTML Web sites will be hardly, if ever, noticeable.

9.4 Comments on the Eye Gaze Tracking Experiment

In addition to their participation in the eye gaze tracking experiment, participants were also asked to provide comments on the experimental protocol, procedure, atmosphere, and/or any other issue related to their experience with the experiment. Overall, the majority of the participants were satisfied with the experiment and commented positively. Many participants mentioned that the experiment was interesting and beneficial to them, as they could see how an actual usability experiment was carried out. However, several aspects of the experiment mentioned by the participants could have also been improved, as follows:

- The setting of the laboratory was made so that the observer was situated on a separate table, but in the same room as the subject (because of the limitations in hardware and wiring). Some participants commented that they felt uncomfortable or they could not browse the Web sites naturally because of the presence of the observer. Some even mentioned that they felt stressful as they were afraid that they might have done something wrong or inappropriate while doing the experiment. There were also a few comments mentioning that the room (approximately six square metres in size) was too small (especially because the equipment took much of the space), too dark, or too hot. However, the lighting condition was set so that the cameras could capture face markers well, as the cameras would not be able to see much contrast in the markers if the light was too bright. Some participants also commented that the eye tracking equipment looked intimidating to them, and it should have been put out of sight, out of mind.

- Because of the difference in the height of each participant, the height of the chair sat on by the participant was adjustable so that his/her whole face was captured by the cameras. The height of the chair was adjusted instead of changing the cameras' angle because the tilt angle of the cameras could not be changed without recalibration. Recalibration of the cameras for each participant was not feasible because it could take up to 24 hours turn-around time for calibration data to be validated by the system provider (for security reasons). The distance between the chair and the cameras was also fixed for the same reason. Therefore, some users felt a bit of discomfort with the height of the chair or the distance between the chair and the monitor provided for them, because different users have different preferences regarding how up/down or close/far from the screen they are comfortable. In addition, as the experiment carried on, some participants often found themselves slouching and therefore the height of the chair was no longer suitable.

- During the screen calibration process, the participants were required to stare at a white dot, which appeared on different parts of the screen, without blinking. They were allowed to blink only when the dot briefly disappeared (before it reappeared). However, several users commented that it was difficult for them not to blink when looking at the dot. In addition, one participant mentioned that the dot (about 1.5 cm in diameter) was so large that he could not help but wander his eyes around the dot. Perhaps a smaller dot could have been more appropriate in this situation; however, the size of the dot could not be customised according to the software used in the experiment. Some participants also had to redo the screen calibration a few times to achieve an acceptable level of accuracy, and they found it tedious to be doing the same thing more than once.

- During the experiment, the use scenarios (tasks) provided for the participants to follow were printed on three sheets of paper, one for each Web site, and placed in front of the keyboard. The font used was Times New Roman (12 points in size), and the tasks were written mostly in a paragraph form (see Appendix 7H). Some users commented that they felt a small degree of discomfort because they thought the font was too small or too cluttered (probably because it was single-spaced), and they had to look down to be able to read. Some participants also suggested that the scenarios should have been written in a bullet-point format in order to catch their attention better and it could have been easier for them to follow. According to the comments, some users also suggest that the use scenarios should be more integrated into the experiment, i.e. in the form of on-screen instructions (e.g. separating the screen into two frames and displaying use scenarios in the top frame while displaying Web sites in the bottom frame, or using separate browser windows or monitors for use scenarios and Web sites). However, some participants preferred the hardcopy, but recommended that it should have been placed at the side of the monitor, instead of on the desk. It was also suggested by some participants that voice instructions could have also been used instead of the written use scenarios.

- The use scenarios for this experiment were aimed at providing the participants with more freedom and flexibility, so that they could browse the Web sites more naturally. Therefore, the tasks were presented as story-telling or imperative sentences without having the users answer specific questions and without any time limit. However, some participants commented that they would prefer the tasks to be presented as questions (similar to those in the Phase One experiment), because they felt that without questions, they were not confident if the goals were accomplished or not. Some participants also preferred time limit to be enforced on each Web site, as they felt easily distracted without official timing.

- Facial expression also plays an important role in the eye gaze tracking process. It was expected that the participant's face remained expressionless during the period of the experiment, otherwise the system would not be able to track facial features accurately (e.g. a person's mouth when smiling looks different than when not smiling). However, some participants said that they found it difficult to maintain a neutral expression during the experiment.

9.5 Analysis of Eye Gaze Point Accuracy

One of the advantages of using eye gaze tracking in usability evaluations is that it can also provide the observer with further information regarding gaze points where the subject is looking while testing the user interface. For this study, the faceLAB eye tracking system provides estimated gaze points as a red circle (approximately 1.5 cm in diameter) superimposed on the video footage of the screen while the user is browsing the Web sites. However, the accuracy of estimated eye gaze points needs to be validated before further investigation can be undertaken. Therefore, the experiment conducted for each participant also incorporated an extra two-minute presentation at the beginning, just before the user viewed the Web sites. This presentation was included as a means for measuring the accuracy of the user's gaze spots estimated by the eye tracking system. During the presentation, 17 different five-figure numbers were shown on different parts of the screen. Each number was presented for four seconds, one after another. The positions of these numbers are shown in Figure 9.7

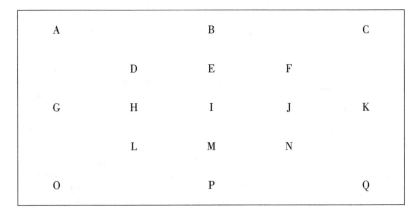

Figure 9.7   Positions of numbers displayed during the presentation

Before the presentation started, the participant was informed about the presentation by the following statement on the screen:

> *Various numbers will appear on different parts of the screen. Each number will appear for four seconds. Please look at each number when it appears and read it out loud. Do NOT click the mouse or press any button on the keyboard.*
>
> *Press Enter to start*

After the participant acknowledged the message by pressing the Enter key, the numbers were presented in random order, while estimated gaze spots were recorded. When the presentation finished, the participant proceeded to browse the Web sites.

According to the video analysis of the presentation, it was found that there were some discrepancies between the estimated gaze points (represented by the red spot) and the actual gaze points (represented by the numbers). It was also found that the misplacements in the Y-axis (up/down) were significantly more dominant than those in the X-axis (left/right). This could be because people's eye opening is wider in the X-axis than the Y-axis; therefore, it is easier for the cameras to detect left-right eye movements with higher accuracy than up-down movements.

Following this observation, the accuracy of the tracking of gaze points was determined by measuring the distance in the Y-axis between the estimated and actual gaze points for each number presented. The distance was measured in centimetres (on a 12-inch monitor), and the sign was also given (plus means that the estimated point is higher than the actual point, minus means the opposite). The displacement value for each number shown on the screen is grouped by position and participant as presented in Tables 9.15 and 9.16, respectively. A mean value is the average of all displacements in consideration, taking into account the sign of each displacement, but a mean absolute value is the average of distances only (no signs).

Therefore, if a mean and its corresponding mean absolute are equal or almost equal in size, the displacements which form that mean must mostly point in the same direction, and vice versa. On the other hand, if these two values differ greatly (i.e. the mean value is close to zero, while the mean absolute is not), it shows that the displacements in question must point up and down sporadically.

Table 9.15 Mean and mean absolute of displacement values (categorised by position)

Position	A	B	C	D	E	F
Mean	-1.19	-1.77	-1.38	-0.91	-0.41	-0.69
Mean Absolute	1.19	1.77	1.38	1.86	1.52	2.02
Position	**G**	**H**	**I**	**J**	**K**	**L**
Mean	-0.61	-0.41	-0.27	-0.13	-0.27	-0.13
Mean Absolute	1.66	1.69	1.77	1.52	1.88	1.52
Position	**M**	**N**	**O**	**P**	**Q**	
Mean	-0.36	0.02	0.94	0.88	0.97	
Mean Absolute	1.30	1.36	0.94	0.88	0.97	

Table 9.16 Mean and mean absolute of displacement values (categorised by participant)

Participant ID	Mean	Mean Absolute	Participant ID	Mean	Mean Absolute	Participant ID	Mean	Mean Absolute
2.1	1.29	1.41	2.14	0.70	0.82	2.27	-3.58	3.58
2.2	-1.23	1.23	2.15	-1.35	2.52	2.28	-1.11	1.11
2.3	Not available*		2.16	-1.70	1.70	2.29	-0.64	0.64
2.4	-2.88	2.88	2.17	-1.47	1.58	2.30	0.64	1.23
2.5	1.11	1.11	2.18	-2.41	2.41	2.31	0.23	1.05
2.6	1.58	1.82	2.19	0.94	0.94	2.32	0.17	0.17
2.7	-0.17	0.29	2.20	-0.47	1.17	2.33	-1.64	1.64
2.8	-0.35	0.58	2.21	1.11	1.11	2.34	-2.94	2.94
2.9	Not available*		2.22	0.88	1.35	2.35	-1.88	1.88
2.10	-0.94	0.94	2.23	0.94	1.41	2.36	2.35	2.47
2.11	Not available*		2.24	0.23	0.35	2.37	-0.11	1.76
2.12	1.17	1.17	2.25	1.70	1.70	2.38	-0.94	1.52
2.13	0.76	0.76	2.26	0.88	1.11	2.39	-3.11	3.11

* Data not available because estimated gaze points during the presentation could not be determined due to technical difficulties, e.g. reflection on glasses

The mean displacement of each screen position is also superimposed on its corresponding position, as shown in Figure 9.8.

A -1.19 (1.19)		B -1.77 (1.77)			C -1.38 (1.38)
	D -0.91 (1.86)	E -0.41 (1.52)	F -0.69 (2.02)		
G -0.61 (1.66)	H -0.41 (1.69)	I -0.27 (1.77)	J -0.13 (1.52)	K -0.27 (1.88)	
	L -0.13 (1.52)	M -0.36 (1.30)	N 0.02 (1.36)		
O 0.94 (0.94)		P 0.88 (0.88)			Q 0.97 (0.97)

Figure 9.8   Positions of displayed numbers and their corresponding mean values of displacements (mean absolute in parentheses)

According to Figure 9.8, it could be seen that the size of mean displacement of each position on the screen differs greatly from its mean absolute (in that the mean is closer to zero), regardless of where it is located, except positions A, B, C, which are located at the top of the screen so all displacements at these positions are negative, and positions O, P, Q, which are located at the bottom of the screen so all displacements at these positions are positive. Hence the mean and mean absolute of these six positions are equal in size. It is also worth noticing that, of all positions on the screen (except the ones in top and bottom rows), the mean values are negative in all but one case (i.e. only position N is positive, albeit very close to zero). Therefore, it could be inferred that overall, the tracking system utilised in the experiment has a tendency to estimate user's gaze point a bit lower than the actual gaze point.

On the other hand, Table 9.16 shows that the size of mean displacement of each participant and the corresponding mean absolute are close in value for most participants. Therefore, it could be inferred that for each participant, the majority of estimated gaze points tend to be displaced in one direction, regardless of their position on the screen. Thus, the accuracy of estimated eye gaze points depends more on each user's calibration than on gaze position on the screen.

According to the accuracy validation results, it could also be inferred that a participant's eye gaze with a smaller mean absolute displacement value was recorded more accurately than that with a larger mean absolute displacement value. However, this is not always the case. Problems arise from various factors during the experiment that make the tracking accuracy changes dramatically over time. From the experiment, it was found that the variation of estimated gaze point accuracy over time and/or across screen areas usually depends on:

- User's eye features, e.g. size (movements of smaller eyes are less apparent than those of larger eyes), colours (eyes with darker iris/pupil are easier to detect), occidental/oriental eyes (oriental eyes are usually flatter and more difficult to detect up/down movements), glasses (reflection of the computer screen or lighting source on glasses makes it more difficult to detect user's eyes)
- User's facial attributes (because the faceLAB system also uses face captures as part of the eye tracking process), e.g. facial features (face with unique and high-contrast features is easier to track), facial expressions during the experiment (smiling, frowning, lip-biting, etc.)
- User's head positions and movements, e.g. movements parallel to the screen (some users tend to move their head across the face of the screen towards the contents they are interested in), movements perpendicular to the screen (some users move their head closer to the screen as the experiment progresses or when they find something interesting or difficult to see or interpret)
- Environmental factors, e.g. lighting condition (also related to camera's brightness/contrast settings), screen size (larger screen provides more accurate tracking)

Therefore, participants with high start-up accuracy could end up with very low accuracy at the end of the experiment, and vice versa. Although the validation process itself was proven to be useful, its effectiveness depends mostly on the eye tracking tool used in the experiment. The nature of eye tracking hardware/software at present, especially the one utilised in this study, could cater for neither constant nor self-adaptive accuracy (discussed in Section 5.5). However, as the technology progresses, it is anticipated that eye tracking systems with either constant or self-adaptive accuracy will become available in the near future.

9.6 Gaze Trails and Look Zones

In the usability evaluation of Web sites, eye gaze trails (created by connecting gaze points that occurred over a period of time) and look zones (specific areas of interest on the screen) can also be used for further qualitative analyses, as discussed in Chapter 5. The analysis of gaze trails is commonly conducted by evaluating the complexity of gaze trails, either subjectively or objectively (with the help of suitable algorithms), or by finding the order in which several objects on the screen were looked at. More complex or pattern-less trails are usually associated with more difficult representations and/or user's confusion. On the other hand, look zones are often analysed by finding the specific amount of time or the number of occurrences that each look zone was looked at during an experiment. These measures can be interpreted in several ways as follows:

- Total fixation duration on Look Zones in terms of frequency: The total amount of fixation duration the user spends on a Look Zone reflects the importance of that Look Zone

- Sequence of fixations: The order in which the user fixates on a design element between Look Zones indicate the efficiency of the arrangements of design elements on the UI
- Percentage of participants on Look Zones: An indicator of how much attention each Look Zone of the UI draws across participants (Tzanidou, 2004)

Not all eye gaze tracking systems readily support the analysis of gaze trails and/or look zones. The faceLAB system utilised in this study does not provide support for either gaze trails or look zones. However, the SDK (Software Development Kit) in several programming languages was provided by the company, so that customisation of the software may be undertaken to accommodate these types of analysis. Nonetheless, software customisation/development is beyond the scope of this research.

Although gaze trails were not provided by the faceLAB system, estimated gaze points were shown on the screen and recorded, as discussed in Section 9.5. Figure 9.9 shows sample screen shots of recorded video footage with overlaid gaze points.

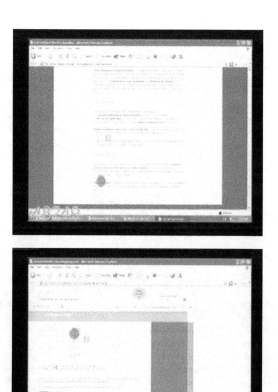

Figure 9.9 Sample screen shots of video footage with overlaid gaze points (filled circles)

Because there is no built-in support for gaze trails in the faceLAB system, one possible alternative is to form imaginary gaze trails by visually combine gaze points over a period of time. However, by analysing the recorded gaze points in detail, it was discovered that another impediment for the analysis of gaze trails in this study, in addition to the lack of software support, is that the gaze points estimated by the system do not provide enough accuracy for this type of analysis because large displacement distances of one to two centimetres (measured on a 12-inch screen[1]) are prevalent and the accuracy is not constant over time (as discussed in Section 9.5). In order for gaze trails to be meaningful, the gaze points that form the trails must be highly accurate, especially in the analysis of Web sites, where there are several small objects on the screen. Displacements of one to two centimetres on a standard PC monitor generate significant errors that make the analysis of gaze points or gaze trails not meaningful because estimated gaze points do not fall on the objects at which the participants were looking at the time of the experiment. In order to increase the accuracy of gaze point tracking, Seeing Machines, the provider of faceLAB, recommends that a video projector be used instead of a standard PC monitor, as follows:

> faceLAB is not intended to be used for precise on-screen gaze tracking with standard PC monitors. If you want to do on-screen gaze tracking experiments, we recommend you use a projector and track the gaze on the large projected image (treating this object as the screen). (Seeing Machines, 2003b, p. 22)

However, a projector screen was not utilised in this study because it would have created unnatural Web browsing behaviours for the participants and hence incurred undesirable complications.

Although the faceLAB eye tracking system does not provide support for look zones within the screen, it promotes the use of look zones outside the screen. This feature is called a "world model," which is an imitation of the environment around the user. These objects around the user, other than the screen, are represented by two- or three-dimensional geometric shapes (e.g. rectangles, spheres). Therefore, it could be inferred that the faceLAB system concentrates on providing support for interactions between users and physical objects around them, instead of focusing on issues regarding look zones inside the screen. However, the interactions between users and items outside the screen are beyond the scope of this study, so the world model feature was not utilised.

9.7 Conclusion

In this chapter, the analyses and results of the second experiment (eye gaze tracking) were presented in detail, including the extraction of eye gaze measurements from raw data and the testing of proposed hypotheses according to the quantitative data gathered. Table 9.17 summarises the hypotheses along with their corresponding status after the tests were performed.

---

[1] The video footage of the Web sites with overlaid gaze points was inevitably compressed and shrunk by the system during the capturing process.

Table 9.17 Summary of research hypotheses (Phase Two)

Hypothesis	Status
H7: Users' eye gaze measures can be affected by Web site version viewed (Flash or HTML).	Not supported
H8: Users' eye gaze measures can be affected by category of Web site version viewed (information, entertainment, or e-commerce).	Weakly supported
H9: Users' eye gaze measures can be determined by gender.	Weakly supported

In addition, qualitative analyses were also performed based on commentary responses from the participants. Results from the qualitative analysis confirm the findings from the first experiment that the Flash version is preferred to the HTML version of Web sites. Comments regarding the eye tracking procedures utilised in the experiment were also summarised and presented. Finally, the proposed method for measuring the accuracy of eye gaze point detection was also realised. The results suggested that the tracking accuracy depended mostly on calibration factors for each individual rather than on position on the screen. Therefore, it could be possible that all the estimated gaze points be transformed to match the real gaze points by utilising a unique transformation formula for each participant. However, the important condition required for the transformation, which is that the displacements must be nearly constant during the tracking period, could not be satisfied because of various factors involved and the limited capability of current technologies. It was also discovered that, although the faceLAB eye tracking system can be used for the usability evaluation of Web sites through quantitative analyses of various eye gaze measures, it may not be the best one because of the lack of support for gaze trails and look zones, which are usually required for further qualitative analyses.

10

Conclusions

10.1 Topics Covered in the Research

There is an old saying that *we never know where we are heading unless we know where we have been.* Therefore, this chapter summarises the materials in this book, so that directions for future research can be determined, in light of what happened before.

At the beginning of this book, an introduction to the field of Human-Computer Interaction was presented. Although HCI as a research field is still young, it has been connecting with several other established fields, ranging from computer science to psychology. With the knowledge contributed by other disciplines and recent research studies, HCI has been growing rapidly and will still do so in the near future. The importance of HCI was emphasised because it is the study of how users communicate with their computers. Through HCI, we can bridge the gap between computer and human territories, which has before been a great barrier preventing the effective use of computers.

Since there are more and more computer users everyday, the development of computer hardware and software has to be adapted towards the needs of people who will be using them. Most computer users demand "ease of use," or in technical terms, "usability." A computer system must be usable by the target audience, or otherwise it would fail to sell. One important aspect of the usability of computer systems is the usability of their user interfaces. It is also the issue concerned by most information technologists because the effective and efficient use of computer software depends largely on this factor. Each and every user interface must be evaluated in one way or another before being distributed to the users. Several methods and techniques for the evaluation of user interfaces were also introduced, with emphasis made on heuristic techniques, including heuristic evaluation and questionnaire. An emerging user observation technique—eye gaze tracking, was also mentioned as a way of getting direct and unbiased information from the users, which can also be used for usability evaluation.

The importance of the Web as a new medium for distributing information to worldwide users was also discussed. Web sites are regarded as user interfaces, and therefore their usability must also be evaluated if effective communication is desired. There are many methods and techniques that can be applied for the usability evaluation of Web sites; many of them are the same as the usability evaluation of traditional user interfaces. Of all the evaluation methods, heuristic evaluation and questionnaire were selected and explored in detail. These two techniques are closely related as they utilise a set of usability heuristics or dimensions, which are criteria that can be used to measure the usability of a Web site. However, the difference is that heuristic evaluation depends on one or more experts to evaluate a Web site based on the selected criteria, while questionnaire depends on users of the Web site to express their opinions regarding the Web site to the evaluator. Therefore, usability heuristics or dimensions are used to select the right questions to ask the users if questionnaires are implemented.

There are two ways of utilising usability heuristics: *non-contingent (traditional)* and *contingent* approaches. For the non-contingent heuristic approach, a same set of usability criteria is used for all Web sites to be evaluated, while the contingent approach selects different sets of dimensions for different Web sites, depending on several factors, such as the purpose of Web sites and target audience characteristics. The advantage of the contingent approach over the traditional approach is that it allows higher flexibility upon the use of usability dimensions. For example, if the non-contingent approach is used, all Web sites to be evaluated by users' survey have to use the same evaluation criteria, and thus the same questions must be presented to the users. This may not be effective because some questions are not relevant to all Web sites in consideration, i.e. only general or superficial questions can be asked. On the other hand, if the contingent heuristic approach is utilised, different Web sites can present different questions to their users, thus the evaluator can select relevant and/or in-depth questions, and therefore gain more valuable information and thorough understanding from survey responses. An example of a contingent heuristic tool (WUCET) was also investigated in great depth, including its conceptual framework and implementation.

In addition to heuristic approaches, user observation techniques are also equally important, as they can also provide effective measures of usability. Eye gaze tracking is one of the emerging user observation techniques, and it was explored in detail in this study. Relevant literature and current technologies regarding this technique were presented comprehensively. Several measures of usability commonly provided by eye tracking systems were also discussed, including saccade/fixation measurements and other measures such as gaze trails and look zones.

Because heuristic approaches and user observation techniques are both powerful, but emphasise different aspects of usability evaluation, it is better to combine both of them to gain synergistic effects than to use any single method alone. Therefore, this study utilised two usability evaluation tools: the WUCET questionnaire (contingent heuristic approach) and the faceLAB eye tracking system (user observation technique).

Research questions and hypotheses were proposed according to the current controversial issue regarding the comparative usability of Flash versus HTML Web sites. During the past few years, Flash technology has become more prevalent than before. It is usual for Web site developers to incorporate new trends like Flash and use them on their Web sites; however, the usability of Flash compared to traditional HTML Web sites was often overlooked, despite the fact that it is very crucial to effective communication with Web site visitors. As a result, several Web site managers have decided to provide both Flash and HTML versions to their users. This practice incurs several disadvantages, including high maintenance costs and increasing discrepancies within the Web sites.

10.2 Summary of Main Results

This study compared the usability of Flash and HTML versions of Web sites by utilising two experiments, corresponding to the two usability evaluation techniques chosen previously. In the first experiment, it was discovered through contingent heuristic questionnaires that users tend to prefer the Flash version of Web sites to the HTML version. This finding was later supported by users' own preferential responses in the second experiment. Therefore, the contingent heuristic approach as represented by the WUCET tool can be considered an effective way of evaluating the usability of Web sites because the results obtained from the questionnaires correspond well to the actual preferences of the users.

Nevertheless, results from the eye gaze tracking experiment do not suggest the difference between Flash and HTML versions of Web sites. However, the differences in eye gaze patterns between gender groups and across Web sites were found. This could be due to the nature of current eye tracking technologies, where the fuzziness of data is still existent, or it could be because the difference is too subtle for the eye tracking method to perceive. This is the reason that usability evaluators should always select more than one technique if time and budget allow, because each usability evaluation technique has its strengths and weaknesses, and thus one technique may uncover the issues that other techniques are unable to.

It was also uncovered in the experiments that user characteristics and Web site purpose can also influence the perceived usability of Web sites. The first experiment suggests that male users tend to prefer Flash version to a greater extent than female users, probably because they enjoy flashy images, animations, and sound effects in Flash Web sites more. It was also found that users with shorter Web/computer experience prefer the Flash version more than users with longer experience, albeit not by much.

The purpose of Web sites was found to influence the usability of Flash and HTML versions, as the Flash version of entertainment Web sites was found to be rated higher in usability than the HTML version to a greater extent than that of e-commerce and information Web sites. Other results also suggest that users with slow Internet connection speed tend to prefer Flash version to a higher degree than users with high speed Internet connection, possibly because Flash Web sites can update contents on specific parts without reloading the whole page, thus providing more flowing browsing experience. Regarding task completion rate, it was also discovered that the Flash version of Web sites is likely to make users complete tasks more accurately than the HTML version, although the difference is only marginal.

Overall, there was strong support for Flash, as a means of producing usable Web sites. However, the research also highlighted some specific issues to be taken into consideration by Web site developers.

10.3 Suggestions for Future Research

A number of facets of the research undertaken indicated directions for future research on the topics covered by this book. More detailed explanations of some phenomena identified in this study, such as differences between gender/experience groups or between Web sites of different categories, can be established by future research concentrating on these issues, in regard to the usability of Web sites. Several aspects of the implementation of contingent heuristic questionnaires can also be improved as discussed in Chapter 8, and replicated for other sets of Web sites.

It is also worth noting that the participants in this study were undergraduate students of Murdoch University. Therefore, the findings in this study are only able to be generalised to parts of the user population with the same characteristics. However, if the results need to be applied to different population groups, such as children or working professionals, it is recommended that further research be undertaken with samples from those population groups, in order to gain results which are more relevant to the groups in consideration.

Regarding the eye gaze tracking technique for the usability evaluation of Web sites, more research studies have to be undertaken, possibly with different tools and/or methodologies. This is because there are many eye tracking systems available, which can support different kinds of measurements. For example, gaze trails and look zones, which may be beneficial for the usability evaluation of Web sites, are not supported by the faceLAB system utilised in this study. In addition, the protocols for the eye gaze tracking experiment in this research provided the participants with a high degree of freedom while browsing the Web sites, as no specific order of tasks or detailed step-by-step use scenarios were forced on the users, because natural eye gaze characteristics, such as saccades and fixations, were desired. However, if future research studies are to be undertaken with emphasis placed on gaze trails and/or look zones, stricter use scenarios may be used so that participants' gaze trails can be compared to the default trails they should follow.

It is also inevitable that further research needs to be conducted with various eye tracking systems, so that the eye gaze tracking technique can be evaluated more effectively, as results from several studies can be compared and comparative performance can be measured, which in turn will benefit practitioners who are seeking suitable eye tracking systems for usability applications.

Overall, this book presents the bridging between theoretical and practical facets of usability evaluation, which are equally important. Theoretical foundations of usability are important because they are the mastermind of any usability testing. However, the practical implementation of evaluation methods and techniques is also crucial to the success of the evaluation, especially at present when there are a large variety of techniques to choose from. Therefore, both academicians and practitioners will benefit from this study, because it emphasises emerging usability evaluation techniques, while it still pays respect to the common aspects of standard usability evaluation.

Appendix 2A

Comparison of four prototyping methods (Vossen and Maguire, 1998)

Prototyping methods	Benefits	Limitations
Paper prototyping	• Potential usability problems can be detected at a very early stage in the design process before any code has been written. • Communication between designers and users is promoted. • Paper prototypes are quick to build / refine, thus enabling rapid design iterations. • Only minimal resources and materials are required.	• Because of their simplicity, paper prototypes do not support the evaluation of fine design detail. • This form of prototype cannot reliably simulate system response times or be used to deliver metric data. • The individual playing the role of the computer must be fully aware of the functionality of the intended system in order to simulate the computer.
Video prototyping	• Usability problems can be detected at a very early stage in the design process (before a commitment to code has been made). • Provides a dynamic simulation of interface elements that can be viewed and commented on by both design teams and intended users. • Minimal resources and materials are required to convey product feel. • The technique can be utilised by those with little or no human factors expertise.	• Staff familiar with the functionality of the intended system are required to create the video prototype. • The method does not actually capture a user interacting with the prototype and lacks the interactive element of other prototyping methods. As such it would perhaps be most suited for demonstration purposes where larger audiences are involved and proof-of-concept is the goal. • Because of the use of simple materials and the lack of interactivity, video prototypes do not support the evaluation of fine design detail or the collection of metrics.
Computer-based prototyping	• This approach permits the swift development of interactive software prototypes. • Prototypes created by this method have a high fidelity with the final product. • The prototypes created under this method also support metric-based evaluations.	• The method requires software development skills. • Although rapid, the method is more time consuming than paper-based approaches. • The resources required are greater due to the use of software and hardware rather than paper and pens. • Due to the greater investment in skills and time there may be some reluctance to 'throw away' a computer-based prototype in contrast to simple paper mock-ups.

Prototyping methods	Benefits	Limitations
Wizard-of-Oz prototyping	• This approach allows usability requirements and issues to be explored at an early stage in the design process, particularly for systems which go beyond readily available technology. While the technique may lack the general applicability of other prototyping approaches it is particularly suited to multimedia and telematics applications. • The member of the design team who plays the wizard can gain valuable insights from the close interaction with end-users.	• The person playing the role of the wizard must master the functionality of the proposed system in order to provide a convincing representation. • This approach requires a higher commitment of resources than other approaches to prototyping such as those that rely on simple paper-based materials. • It may be difficult to carry this out effectively in situations where there is a large graphic element in the interface.

Appendix 2B
Ten usability heuristics (Nielsen, 1994a)

1. Visibility of system status: The system should always keep users informed about what is going on, through appropriate feedback within reasonable time.
2. Match between system and the real: The system should speak the users' language, with words, phrases and concepts familiar to the user, rather than system-oriented terms. Follow real-world conventions, making information appear in a natural and logical order.
3. User control and freedom: Users often choose system functions by mistake and will need a clearly marked "emergency exit" to leave the unwanted state without having to go through an extended dialogue. Support undo and redo.
4. Consistency and standards: Users should not have to wonder whether different words, situations, or actions mean the same thing. Follow platform conventions.
5. Error prevention: Even better than good error messages is a careful design which prevents a problem from occurring in the first place.
6. Recognition rather than recall: Make objects, actions, and options visible. The user should not have to remember information from one part of the dialogue to another. Instructions for use of the system should be visible or easily retrievable whenever appropriate.
7. Flexibility and efficiency of use: Accelerators—unseen by the novice user— may often speed up the interaction for the expert user such that the system can cater to both inexperienced and experienced users. Allow users to tailor frequent actions.
8. Aesthetic and minimalist design: Dialogues should not contain information which is irrelevant or rarely needed. Every extra unit of information in a dialogue competes with the relevant units of information and diminishes their relative visibility.
9. Help users recognize, diagnose, and recover from errors: Error messages should be expressed in plain language (no codes), precisely indicate the problem, and constructively suggest a solution.
10. Help and documentation: Even though it is better if the system can be used without documentation, it may be necessary to provide help and documentation. Any such information should be easy to search, focused on the user's task, list concrete steps to be carried out, and not be too large.

Appendix 2C
Web site evaluation checklist (Gaffney, 1998)

	Compliance		
	Always	**Sometimes**	**Never**
Navigation			
There is a clear indication of the current location	☐	☐	☐
There is a clearly-identified link to the Home page	☐	☐	☐
All major parts of the site are accessible from the Home page	☐	☐	☐
If necessary, a site map is available	☐	☐	☐
Site structure is simple, with no unnecessary levels	☐	☐	☐
If necessary, an easy-to-use Search function is available	☐	☐	☐
Functionality			
All functionality is clearly labelled	☐	☐	☐
All necessary functionality is available without leaving the site	☐	☐	☐
No unnecessary plug-ins are used	☐	☐	☐
Control			
The user can cancel all operations	☐	☐	☐
There is a clear exit point on every page	☐	☐	☐
Page size is less than 50Kb/page	☐	☐	☐
All graphic links are also available as text links	☐	☐	☐
The site supports the user's workflow	☐	☐	☐
All appropriate browsers are supported	☐	☐	☐
Language			
The language used is simple	☐	☐	☐
Jargon is avoided	☐	☐	☐
Feedback			
It is always clear what is happening on the site	☐	☐	☐
Users can receive email feedback if necessary	☐	☐	☐
All feedback is prompt	☐	☐	☐
Users are informed if a plug-in or browser version is required	☐	☐	☐
Users can give feedback via email or a feedback form	☐	☐	☐
If necessary, online help is available	☐	☐	☐
Consistency			
Only one word or term is used to describe any item	☐	☐	☐
Links match titles of the pages to which they refer	☐	☐	☐
Standard colours are used for links and visited links	☐	☐	☐
Terminology is consistent with general web usage	☐	☐	☐
Error prevention and correction			
Errors do not occur unnecessarily	☐	☐	☐
Error messages are in plain language	☐	☐	☐
Error messages describe what action is necessary	☐	☐	☐
Error messages provide a clear exit point	☐	☐	☐
Error messages provide contact details for assistance	☐	☐	☐
Visual clarity			
The layout is clear	☐	☐	☐
There is sufficient 'white space'	☐	☐	☐
All images have ALT text assigned	☐	☐	☐
Unnecessary animation is avoided	☐	☐	☐

Appendix 3A
How to conduct a heuristic evaluation (Xerox, 1996)

Getting Ready (Project Lead activities)
1. Identify and define the usability principles (heuristics) that you will use to evaluate the user interface system.
2. Select your evaluation team. Identify three to five usability professionals to examine the system on an individual basis.
3. Schedule locations, days, and times for each usability professional to assess the system.
4. Prepare or compile materials that will enable the evaluators to become familiar with the purpose of the system and of its users. These materials can include: audience analysis, system specification, user tasks, use case scenarios, etc. Distribute these materials to the evaluators.
5. Design your evaluation and notetaking strategy. Are you are going to evaluate the system on an individual or group basis? Are you are going to assign a common notetaker or ask each individual to take his or her own notes?

Evaluating the system (Evaluator activities)
1. Experiment with and establish a feel for the scope of the system.
2. Review the materials provided to familiarize yourself with the system design. Perform the user actions that you feel would be taken to perform the user tasks.
3. Identify and list any areas of the system that you feel are counter to the heuristics. List all of the concerns that you note, including what seem to be duplicates. Be sure to clearly describe what you find, including where in the system it was found.

Analyzing the results (group activity)
1. Review each of the concerns noted by each of the evaluators. Make sure that each concern is clearly understood by all evaluators.
2. Develop an affinity diagram that groups similar concerns.
3. Evaluate and judge each concern for its compliance with your defined heuristic.
4. Assign an severity level for each grouped concern based on the impact to the end user.
5. Determine recommendations to fix the problem. Make sure each recommendation links the heuristic and a design principle.

Reporting the results (Team Leader activity)
1. Compile the results of the group meeting of the evaluators. Each problem should have a severity code, a link to a design principle, an explanation of the usability issue, and a recommendation.
2. Report all sources, purposes, techniques, procedures, and findings in a format that is easy to read and understand. You may decide to organize you findings by design principle (heuristic). Be sure to note the positive attributes of the system or interface.

3. Make sure the report includes a mechanism for the Project Team Lead to report back on how the information was used by the development team.
4. Have your report reviewed by another team member, and approved by team coach.

Debriefing (Team Leader activity)
1. Schedule a time and location for your oral presentation if required by the customer.
2. Focus on the major usability concerns and possible solutions.
3. Highlight the positive attributes concerning the design.
4. Follow up with the Project Team Lead as necessary.

Severity Rating Scales
You can decide to use either of these severity rating scale, or develop you own to suit the project needs.

Five-point rating scale
1. Cosmetic, will not affect the usability of the system, fix if possible.
2. Minor, users can easily work around the problem, fixing this should be given low priority.
3. Medium, users stumble over the problem, but quickly adapt to it, fixing this should be given medium priority
4. Major, users have difficulty, but are able to find workarounds, fixing this should be mandatory before the system is launched. If the problem cannot be fixed before launch, ensure that the documentation clearly shows the user a workaround
5. Catastrophic, users are unable to do their work, fixing this is mandatory

Three-point scale
1. Low: cosmetic or minor, causes minimal difficulty
2. Moderate: causes some problems to doing work or causes the user to stumble, but recovery is possible.
3. High: effectively prevents the user from doing work, the user will fail or have extreme difficulty.

Appendix 3B
Quick review heuristic feedback (Naughton, 1995)

This dialog's interface design:	How critical is this requirement?		
1. language and phrases familiar to user	___ Low	___ Medium	___ High
2. organizes screen information in a natural and logical order	___ Low	___ Medium	___ High
3. facilitates users decision making and task processing	___ Low	___ Medium	___ High
4. provides an easy exit for the user	___ Low	___ Medium	___ High
5. supports undo and redo functionality	___ Low	___ Medium	___ High
6. prevents user error	___ Low	___ Medium	___ High
7. provides error messages that indicate the error and recovery processes	___ Low	___ Medium	___ High
8. provides visual cues for easy task processing	___ Low	___ Medium	___ High
9. allows swift and easy processing for experienced users while supporting novice users	___ Low	___ Medium	___ High
10. organizes rarely used dialog information to promote visibility of all important dialog elements	___ Low	___ Medium	___ High
11. provides visual help cues that are easily accessed and consistent (help button)	___ Low	___ Medium	___ High
12. is quick and easy to use	___ Low	___ Medium	___ High
13. provides user feedback and system status when needed	___ Low	___ Medium	___ High
14. is designed to be visually pleasing to the user	___ Low	___ Medium	___ High
15. allows for rapid, accurate and complete task processing	___ Low	___ Medium	___ High
16. provides security features to protect personal or private information	___ Low	___ Medium	___ High
17. meets physical handicap requirements	___ Low	___ Medium	___ High
18. is consistent with other dialogs designed for this system	___ Low	___ Medium	___ High
19. works well within the specific processing environment conditions	___ Low	___ Medium	___ High

Appendix 4A
Contingency table prioritisations (Dunstan, 2003, pp. 237-245)

Usability Dimension	Age			
	General	Middle-Aged	Old	Young
Adherence to Conventions/Standards	3.5	3.8	4.6	2.1
Attractiveness/Annoyance	3.6	4.2	2.1	4.6
Clarity/Presentation	3.8	3.6	4.6	3.3
Content	4.2	4.5	3.7	4.4
Customisability	3.8	4.0	3.2	4.2
Download Speed	3.2	2.8	2.1	4.6
Ease of downloads	3.5	4.2	2.2	4.0
Error Reduction/Recovery	3.3	3.2	4.6	2.0
H/W and S/W requirements	3.6	2.8	3.8	4.2
Help/Documentation	3.5	4.1	4.6	1.7
Hyperlinks	4.1	4.6	3.3	4.4
Integrity/Ethics	3.3	3.8	4.6	1.5
Interaction Opportunities	3.3	3.2	2.1	4.5
Navigation support	3.4	3.4	4.6	2.2
Reliability	3.1	4.0	2.2	3.2
Search facilities	3.8	4.0	3.3	4.0

Usability Dimension	Culture		
	Asian	General	Western
Adherence to Conventions/Standards	4.2	3.7	3.2
Attractiveness/Annoyance	2.6	2.9	3.2
Clarity/Presentation	4.4	4.4	4.4
Content	3.1	3.9	4.7
Customisability	4.2	3.4	2.6
Download Speed	4.8	3.9	2.9
Ease of downloads	2.8	2.8	2.8
Error Reduction/Recovery	3.0	2.5	1.9
H/W and S/W requirements	3.5	3.5	3.5
Help/Documentation	2.2	2.2	2.2
Hyperlinks	3.4	3.3	3.2
Integrity/Ethics	4.4	4.0	3.6
Interaction Opportunities	3.1	3.1	3.1
Navigation support	2.7	2.4	2.1
Reliability	3.4	3.4	3.4
Search facilities	4.5	4.5	4.5

Usability Dimension	Disability			
	Cognitive	Hearing	None	Visual
Adherence to Conventions/Standards	4.8	3.1	2.2	4.8
Attractiveness/Annoyance	4.7	3.2	4.3	3.6
Clarity/Presentation	4.8	4.3	3.2	4.8
Content	1.2	4.1	4.1	3.7
Customisability	4.8	4.8	2.2	4.5
Download Speed	1.1	4.5	2.8	4.3
Ease of downloads	4.8	4.2	2.9	4.2
Error Reduction/Recovery	4.8	4.0	2.6	3.6
H/W and S/W requirements	3.9	4.0	3.1	4.0
Help/Documentation	4.0	4.0	2.6	4.3
Hyperlinks	2.7	2.8	4.2	2.8
Integrity/Ethics	2.9	3.2	3.1	2.1
Interaction Opportunities	1.2	3.7	2.9	2.3
Navigation support	4.3	2.2	2.4	4.0
Reliability	2.2	3.3	3.2	3.3
Search facilities	1.5	3.7	3.6	3.7

Usability Dimension	Education			
	General	Primary	Secondary	Tertiary/ Post
Adherence to Conventions/Standards	3.1	3.6	2.4	3.4
Attractiveness/Annoyance	3.8	4.1	4.2	3.2
Clarity/Presentation	4.2	4.6	3.6	4.4
Content	4.4	4.0	4.5	4.7
Customisability	3.0	2.1	2.8	4.0
Download Speed	3.3	3.8	3.2	2.9
Ease of downloads	3.6	4.0	4.0	2.8
Error Reduction/Recovery	3.7	4.8	4.4	1.8
H/W and S/W requirements	3.5	4.2	2.8	3.5
Help/Documentation	3.5	4.8	4.0	1.8
Hyperlinks	3.8	3.2	3.9	4.4
Integrity/Ethics	2.9	1.5	2.4	4.8
Interaction Opportunities	3.7	4.5	3.6	3.1
Navigation support	3.7	4.8	4.4	1.8
Reliability	3.2	3.2	2.9	3.4
Search facilities	3.6	3.1	3.2	4.5

Usability Dimension	WWW/IT Experience		
	General	High	Low
Adherence to Conventions/Standards	3.8	3.4	4.1
Attractiveness/Annoyance	3.0	2.6	3.4
Clarity/Presentation	4.4	4.4	4.4
Content	4.3	4.7	3.8
Customisability	3.6	3.6	3.5
Download Speed	3.1	3.8	2.4
Ease of downloads	4.0	3.5	4.4
Error Reduction/Recovery	3.3	1.8	4.8
H/W and S/W requirements	2.6	3.5	1.6
Help/Documentation	2.7	0.8	4.6
Hyperlinks	4.1	4.8	3.3
Integrity/Ethics	2.5	2.4	2.6
Interaction Opportunities	3.2	4.4	2.0
Navigation support	3.2	1.8	4.6
Reliability	4.2	4.3	4.1
Search facilities	3.6	4.5	2.7

Usability Dimension	Site Purpose*					
	CO	EN	IN	SE	EC	MA
Adherence to Conventions/Standards	4.6	2.3	3.7	3.6	3.9	3.2
Attractiveness/Annoyance	2.5	4.8	3.5	2.6	4.6	4.8
Clarity/Presentation	3.4	4.3	4.8	3.8	3.8	4.8
Content	2.8	3.9	4.9	4.2	4.0	3.4
Customisability	3.4	3.3	2.2	1.9	2.5	1.6
Download Speed	4.8	4.5	4.0	4.0	4.6	4.4
Ease of downloads	3.9	4.4	2.7	1.4	2.4	2.3
Error Reduction/Recovery	2.8	2.7	3.0	2.6	3.9	1.3
H/W and S/W requirements	3.0	4.6	1.8	2.7	4.0	4.8
Help/Documentation	2.2	1.3	3.4	3.8	3.4	2.2
Hyperlinks	4.1	4.0	4.8	4.0	4.0	4.4
Integrity/Ethics	2.2	3.8	4.0	4.0	4.8	4.4
Interaction Opportunities	4.8	4.1	2.0	2.5	4.4	4.2
Navigation support	4.2	3.2	3.6	3.1	2.6	2.3
Reliability	3.8	2.8	3.1	4.2	4.5	3.7
Search facilities	3.5	4.0	4.8	4.4	4.8	4.4

* CO = Communication
  EN = Entertainment
  IN = Information
  SE = Services
  EC = E-Commerce
  MA = Marketing

Appendix 4B
WUCET question pool (Dunstan, 2003, pp. 260-261)

Usability Dimension	Description	Questions (unfavourable in italics)
a. Content	usefulness; relevance; accuracy; truthfulness; completeness; currency	1. The content of this web site is useful for its intended purpose and audience. 2. *This web site is not accurate or truthful with the information presented.* 3. Information presented at this site is complete.
b. Hyperlinks	quantity; quality; relevance; currency (dangling?)	1. The hyperlinks on this web site are adequate but not overwhelming. 2. *The words used to describe the hyperlink (i.e. underlined) are vague.* 3. The hyperlinks are all current.
c. Clarity / Presentation	simplicity; elegance; layout structure; use of graphics; readability	1. This web site is easily readable and relatively easy to understand. 2. The layout of this web site lends itself to good planning of activities. 3. This web site is not cluttered with unnecessary diagrams/graphics/etc.
d. Adherence to Conventions/ Standards	to the extent that they apply to the site purpose	1. *The layout of this web site does not adhere to standards/conventions.* 2. *Adherence to standards means this site is not very innovative or attractive.* 3. This web site adheres to the purposes it was designed for.
e. Navigation Support	structured layout; site map; navigation buttons; search; links; frames	1. It is easy to understand where you are on this web site. 2. *The use of panels, frames or dedicated areas to facilitate navigation is not very useful.* 3. The site map, or overview diagram is effective.
f. Search Facilities	functionality; utility	1. This site enables you to search on its content. 2. Searching on this site yields good (and relevant) results. 3. *The way searches are structured is not very useful.*
g. Attractiveness / Annoyance	images; video; sounds; animations; banners; creativity; innovations	1. This web site is attractive. 2. *This web site is annoying.* 3. Animations, blinking effects, music, banners, etc support the purpose of this web site.
h. Interaction Opportunities	creativity; functionality; utility	1. There are ample opportunities to interact with this web site. 2. *Interactions that this web site allows do not really support its purpose.* 3. The types of interactions permitted are innovative.
i. Error Reduction / Recovery	design to limit errors; undo facility	1. The design of this web site reduces mistakes in user understanding of content. 2. *This web site does not allow a user to undo an error.* 3. *It is easy to make navigation errors in this site.*

Usability Dimension	Description	Questions (unfavourable in italics)
j. Help / Documentation	availability; utility	1. You are able to find a help page, or help-related page quite easily. 2. *Users will need assistance in using this web site.* 3. The help documentation is relevant and effective to the workings of this web site.
k. Download Speed	number and format of graphics; thumbnails; progressive build up	1. The time to download this web site is adequate, given the speed of your Internet connection. 2. *Thumbnails provided do not make much difference to the download speed of this web site.* 3. The progressive build up to this web site, in terms of graphics downloads is effective.
l. H/W and S/W Requirements	restrictions; reliance on downloads; needing latest browser version	1. *I have to use the latest version of the browser to get the most out of this site.* 2. This web site does not require special downloads, easing the burden on my machine. 3. The machine and browser you are currently using provides for easy browsing of this site.
m. Reliability	does server go down often	1. *The server of this web-site is down or busy making browsing very slow or not effective.* 2. There have been no interruptions (network-related) in using this web site. 3. *I have frequently found problems accessing this web site.*
n. Customisability	user model / profile; cookies for user attributes	1. This web site can conform to particular user characteristics, i.e. languages, cultures. 2. *There are only limited facilities to tailor this web site to different types of users.* 3. This web site can save user attributes (i.e. cookies), and use them in future browsing sessions.
o. Ease of Downloads	range of material available; format of files	1. There are lots of useful downloads available on this web site. 2. Downloads are relatively easy to perform on this web site. 3. File sizes at this web site are not too large, enabling quicker access.
p. Integrity / Ethics	security (e.g. use of credit card no / email address); race / gender treatment	1. I trust this web site enough to provide my Credit Card number, or personal information. 2. *There is poor consideration for race or gender groups on this web site.* 3. This web site is unlikely to offend anyone.

Appendix 4C
List of Web usability criteria (Hassan and Li, 2001)

Category/ Factor	Subcategory	Criteria	
		Objective	**Subjective**
1. Screen design	Space allocation	• Position of menu/ list of contents on screen (left or right hand side of the screen) • Location of menu bar/ tools bar/ navigation bar (at the top or bottom of the screen)	• Proper allocation of screen spaces for content display, menu bar, list of contents, and advertisement
	Choice of colour	• Sharp colour contrast between background and foreground • Use of colour to differentiate functional area (e.g. tool bar, menu bar and list of contents) with content display area • Use of conservative colour • Use of light colour (white/yellow) colour for background	• Minimal use of colour except for photos and graphics
	Readability	• Use a mixture of upper and lower case for text • Use of all capital letters for captions and labels • Different text sizes to differentiate between titles, headings and texts	• Use of fonts that are easy to read
	Scannability	• Clear titles for each pages • Clear headings, sub headings for text/ document • Short paragraphs (not more than 6 sentences) • Use of typography and skimming layout, for example, bold fonts and highlighted words	-
2. Content	Scope	• Suitable language for audience • Publication and press release • Archive of previously published materials	• Breadth of subject coverage • Depth of subject coverage • Intrinsic value of information
	Accuracy	-	• High quality writing, for example, good grammar and no spelling and typographical error • Separation between informational and opinion content

Category/ Factor	Subcategory	Criteria	
		Objective	Subjective
	Authority	• Name of text or documents' authors • Positions or affiliations of text or documents' authors • References or sources of text/ document • Background information of institution/ organisation/ owner of the site i.e. name, address, phone number and email address • Copyright holder statement	-
	Currency	• Resource date • Page revision date	-
	Uniqueness	• Output/ print format as alternative to HTML format • Viewing format other than HTML, for example, PDF and slides • Choices of language for multi-ethnic audience • Choices of media type for information, for example, text only, audio or video • Hit counter • Information or warnings on file type and size for downloading	-
	Linkages	• Links to other relevant sites • Links to state and local branches • Links to supporting or sponsoring organisations	-
3. Accessibility	Loading speed	-	• Acceptable loading time (10 – 20 seconds)
	Browser compatibility	• Compatible contents for all main browsers (Netscape and Microsoft Explorer) • Compatible contents between different versions of the same browser	-
	Search facility	• Search facility for medium and large web sites	-
	Web site accessibility	• Links available in other relevant web sites	-
4. Navigation	-	• Menu/ list of contents in the main page • Menu/ list of contents in every page • Links to anywhere from anywhere within the site • Minimal number of links to arrive at a particular information • Use of both graphics and textbased menu • Accurate and up-to-date links • Use of sitemap	• Appropriate number of sections/ categories of contents (not more than 7)

Category/ Factor	Subcategory	Criteria	
		Objective	Subjective
5. Media use	Audio	• Control features for audio where appropriate , for example, replay, control volume and turn off	• Use of audio to suit context, for example, instruction, speeches, and songs
	Graphics and images	• Use of graphics or/and images for emphasis • Use of graphics or/and images to attract attention • Labelling of all graphics and images • Use of thumbnails to display photos	• Minimal use of cosmetic graphics and images
	Animation and video	• Use of animation and video as guides to users • Control features for animation and video where appropriate, for example, repeat, slow down, turn off • Avoidance of looping animation to prevent users' distraction	• Relevant use of moving pictures media i.e. animation and video
6. Interactivity	-	• Features for users' feedback about the site, for example, web master's email address and on-line form • Features for sharing views and discussions, for example, e-forum, net conference and net chatting	-
7. Consistency	-	• Consistent page layout, for example, screen size for content display, banners, and menu bar. • Consistent use of text in terms of its type, font size and colour. • Consistent use of navigational aids, for example, menu bar, buttons and links in terms of graphics metaphor, size and colour.	-

Appendix 5A
Glossary of eye tracking terms

Fixation

A fixation occurs when the eye is "stationary" between saccades and it is convenient to assume that the area imaged on to the fovea (or very near to the fovea) during a fixation is being visually attended to by the observer. Fixations differ in their duration but tend to be about 200-300ms, although much longer fixations can occur. The length of fixations is an important research topic in itself as it relates to the visual information to which the observer is attending as well as to his/her cognitive state. Precisely when a fixation starts and ends is itself a matter of research interest as the recorded fixation length is itself somewhat related to the temporal sampling rate of the eye movement recording technique being used. (Applied Vision Research Unit, 2004)

LookZone

A LookZone is a point or multiple points on a web site that the site owner wants to know has or hasn't been looked at. It might be an advert for a particular product or, in the case of a search engine, a sponsored link. Multiple subject analysis is also an option, working out the average amount of time or percentage time a group of subjects spent in these predefined areas. (Barber, Janes, and Boyland, 2004)

PERCLOS

PERCLOS is the percentage of eyelid closure over the pupil over time and reflects slow eyelid closures ("droops") rather than blinks. A PERCLOS drowsiness metric was established in a 1994 driving simulator study as the proportion of time in a minute that the eyes are at least 80 percent closed. (Federal Highway Administration, 1998)

Saccade

A saccade is a rapid eye movement (a jump) which is usually conjugate (i.e. both eyes move together in the same direction) and under voluntary control. Broadly speaking the purpose of these movements is to move the eyes such that images of particular areas of the visual world fall onto the fovea. Saccades are therefore a major instrument of selective visual attention. It is often convenient (but somewhat inaccurate) to consider both that a saccadic eye movement always occurs in a straight line and also that we do not "see" during these movements. We can therefore simply consider that we often see the world by means of a series of saccadic jumps from one area to another, interspersed with fixations. Note, however, that these are oversimplifications. (Applied Vision Research Unit, 2004)

Appendix 6A
Examples of well-known Web sites offering both Flash and HTML versions to the users

Entertainment Web sites:

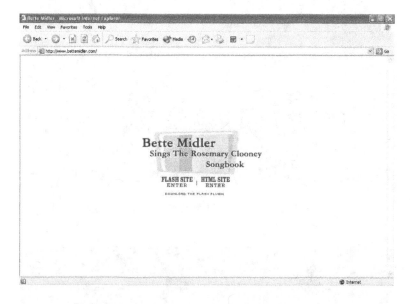

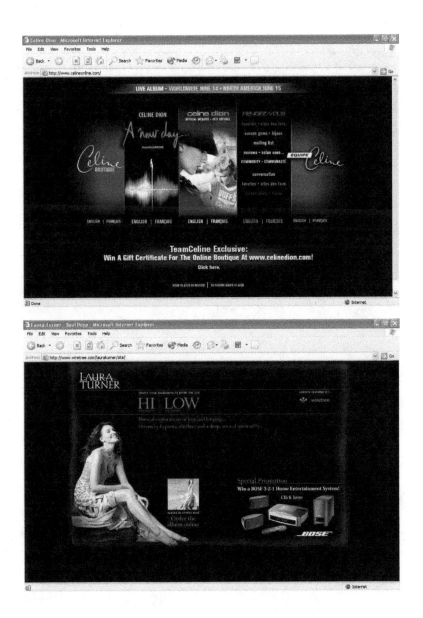

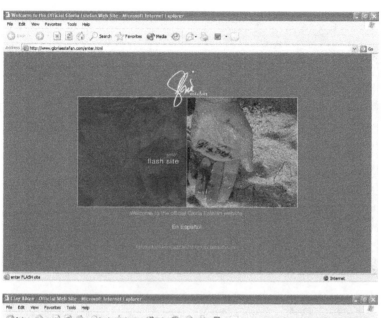

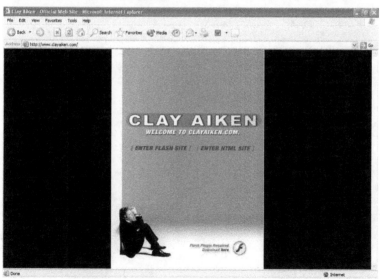

199

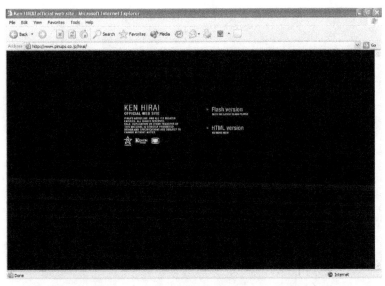

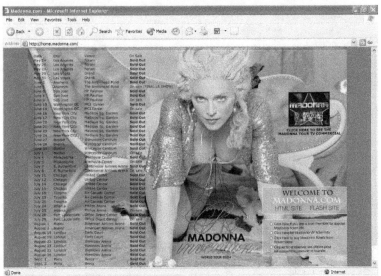

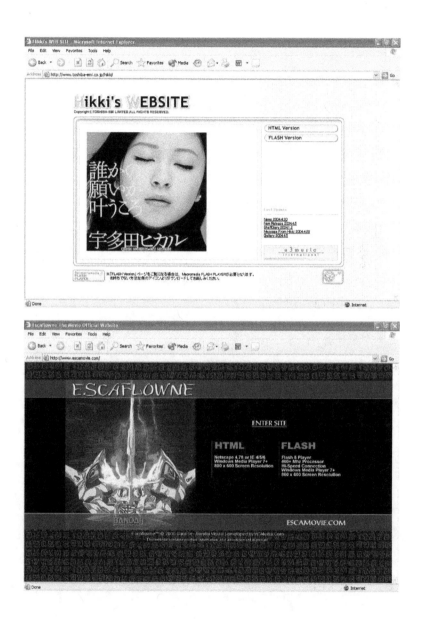

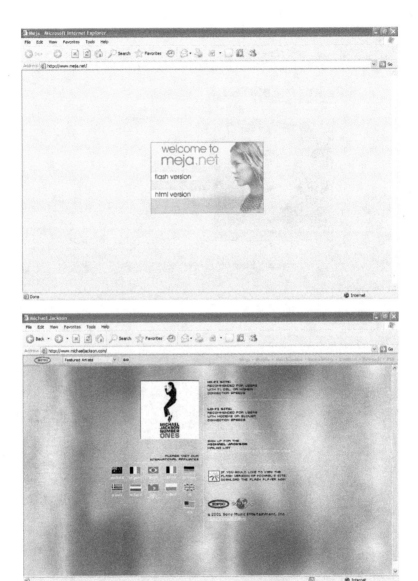

E-Commerce Web sites:

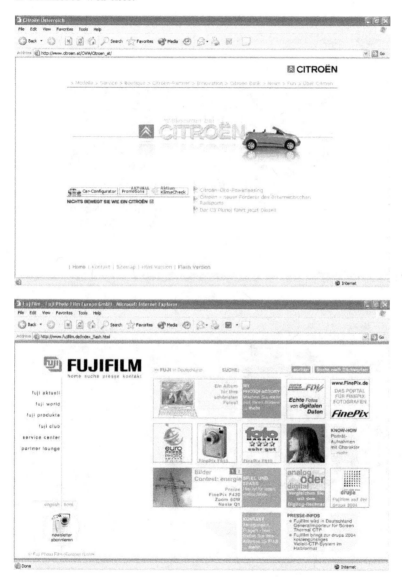

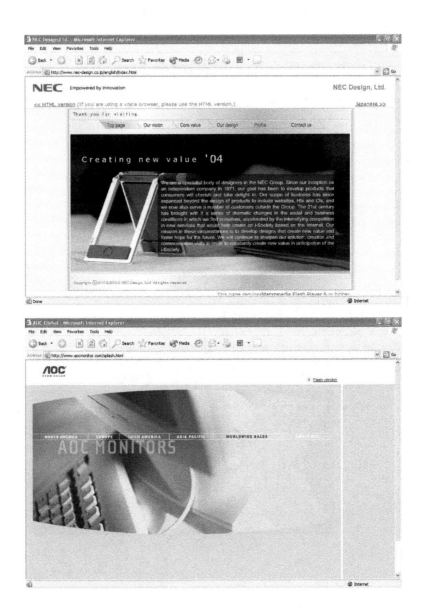

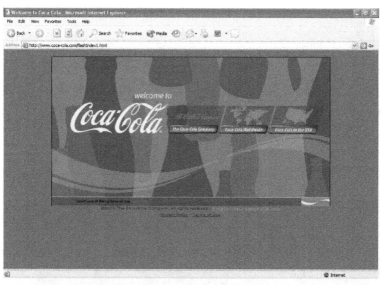

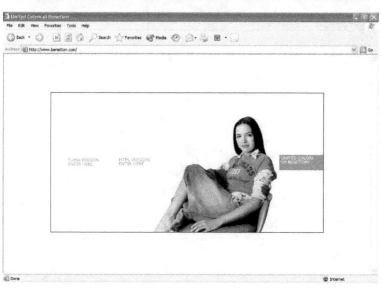

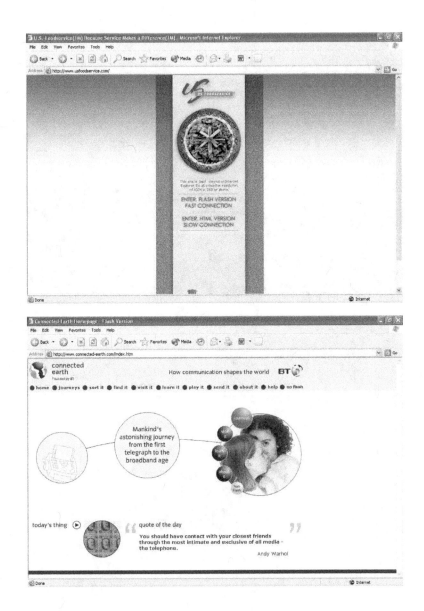

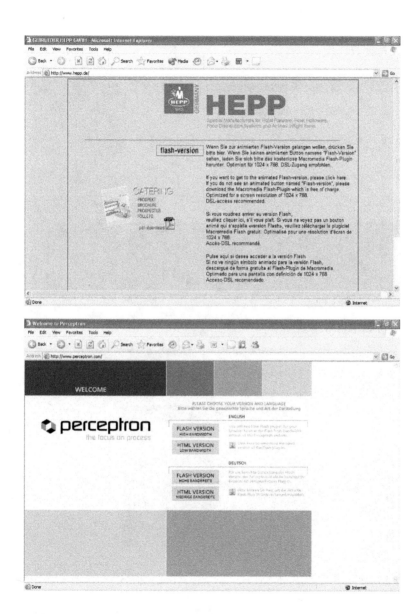

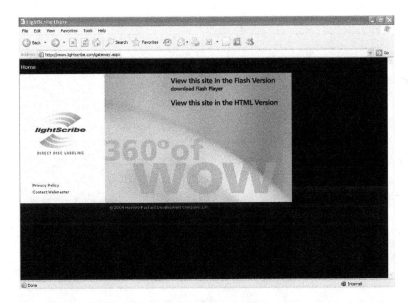

Information Web sites:

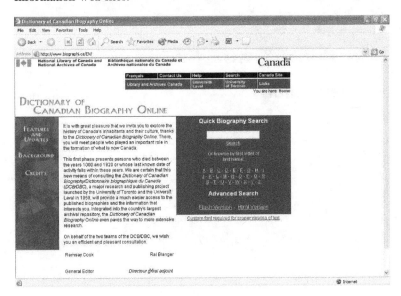

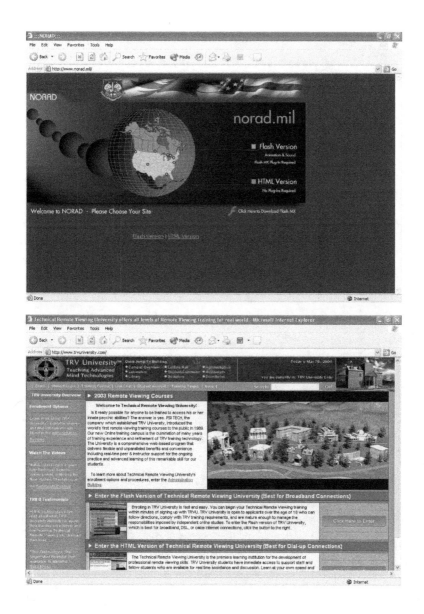

209

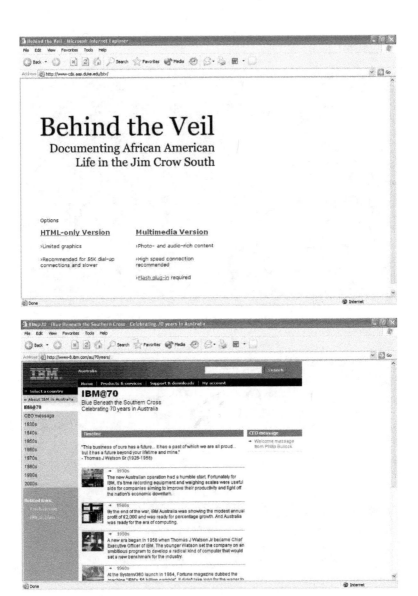

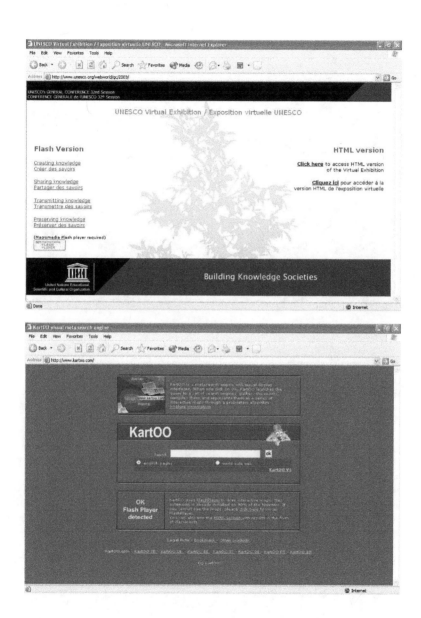

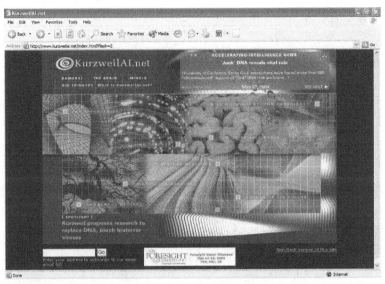

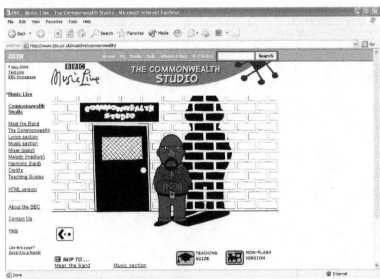

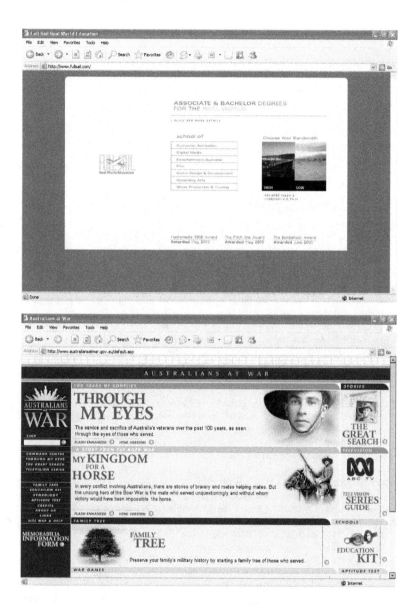

Appendix 7A
Detailed procedures for the pilot study of usability survey

In this survey, you will be asked to find out some information from six different web sites.

Please note that you are not required to provide the information you have found, but only your evaluation of how easy or difficult it was for you to find the information.

Once you click the link in the e-mail you receive after you enroll, you will be directed to the first page of the survey. When you are ready to begin, click "next."

Background Information
Please answer all questions provided. After you have completed the background information, click "next." You will be taken to Part A of the survey.

Part A: "Full Sail" Web Site
Click on the link to the "Full Sail" web site, which will open in a new browser window. (Note: If the site is not accessible for any reason, please indicate so in the survey window.) When you are ready to begin, click the "Start" button of the timer at the top and then do the following tasks:
1. Find out what courses are being offered in the Game Design and Development degree.
2. Find out the career prospects for the program.
3. Find out the prerequisites for admission to Full Sail.
4. Find out where Full Sail is located. (Hint: check out the "Visit Full Sail" section)

Once you finish these tasks, click the "Stop" button of the timer and note the time you used (in seconds). Now go back to the survey window, answer the questions, and evaluate the site by rating the statements provided. If you are unsure how to rate some statements, you may revisit the web site and browse around as freely as you like. Once you have answered all questions, click "next."

Part B: "Australians At War" Web Site
Click on the link to the "Australians At War" web site, which will open in a new browser window. (Note: If the site is not accessible for any reason, please indicate so in the survey window.) When you are ready to begin, click the "Start" button of the timer at the top and then do the following tasks:
1. Find out on what date Britain declared World War I.
2. Find out how many Australians gave their lives during World War II.
3. Find out how many countries contributed in the Korean War.
4. Find out how many Australians served in the Vietnam War.

Once you finish these tasks, click the "Stop" button of the timer and note the time you used (in seconds). Now go back to the survey window, answer questions, and evaluate the site by rating the statements provided. If you are unsure how to rate some statements, you may revisit the web site and browse around as freely as you like. Once you have answered all questions, click "next."

Part C: "Escaflowne" Web Site
Click on the link to the "Escaflowne" web site, which will open in a new browser window. (Note: If the site is not accessible for any reason, please indicate so in the survey window.) When you are ready to begin, click the "Start" button of the timer at the top and then do the following tasks:

1. Check out the storyline of *Escaflowne The Movie* and find out on what planet this story is set.
2. Check out the characters and find out who Hitomi and Van are.
3. Find out what is contained in Disk 3 of the Escaflowne Ultimate Edition DVD Box Set. (Hint: check out the "Home Video" section)

Once you finish these tasks, click the "Stop" button of the timer and note the time you used (in seconds). Now go back to the survey window, answer the questions, and evaluate the site by rating the statements provided. If you are unsure how to rate some statements, you may revisit the web site and browse around as freely as you like. Once you have answered all questions, click "next."

Part D: "Disturbed" Web Site
Click on the link to the "Disturbed" web site, which will open in a new browser window. (Note: If the site is not accessible for any reason, please indicate so in the survey window.) When you are ready to begin, click the "Start" button of the timer at the top and then do the following tasks:

1. Find out who are the members of Disturbed. (Hint: check out the "About" section)
2. Find out the release date of their debut album entitled *The Sickness*.
3. Check out their tour dates and find out where they are performing this month.

Once you finish these tasks, click the "Stop" button of the timer and note the time you used (in seconds). Now go back to the survey window, answer the questions, and evaluate the site by rating the statements provided. If you are unsure how to rate some statements, you may revisit the web site and browse around as freely as you like. Once you have answered all questions, click "next."

Part E: "Chronicle Books" Web Site
Click on the link to the "Chronicle Books" web site, which will open in a new browser window. (Note: If the site is not accessible for any reason, please indicate so in the survey window.) When you are ready to begin, click the "Start" button of the timer at the top and then do the following tasks:

1. Find out which books have just been released. (Hint: check out "What's Hot")
2. Try adding any new release book to your shopping cart.
3. Use the "Gift Finder" to find a book for your mother for her birthday. She loves cooking. Choose one book and add to your shopping cart.
4. Find out the customer service phone number of Chronicle Books. (Hint: check out the "Information" section)

Once you finish these tasks, click the "Stop" button of the timer and note the time you used (in seconds). Now go back to the survey window, answer the questions, and evaluate the site by rating the statements provided. If you are unsure how to rate some statements, you may revisit the web site and browse around as freely as you like. Once you have answered all questions, click "next."

Part F: "Perceptron" Web Site
Click on the link to the "Perceptron" web site, which will open in a new browser window. (Note: If the site is not accessible for any reason, please indicate so in the survey window.) When you are ready to begin, click the "Start" button of the timer at the top and then do the following tasks:
1. Find out in what year Perceptron was founded. (Hint: check out the "Company" section)
2. Find out what is Perceptron's AutoScan system.
3. Find out the address and phone number of Perceptron's Japan regional office.

Once you finish these tasks, click the "Stop" button of the timer and note the time you used (in seconds). Now go back to the survey window, answer the questions, and evaluate the site by rating the statements provided. If you are unsure how to rate some statements, you may revisit the web site and browse around as freely as you like. Once you have answered all questions, click "next."

Final Step
If you are satisfied with all your answers, click the "submit" button and wait for the confirmation message. Otherwise, you can go back and check or edit your answers by clicking "prev." After you make changes to your answers, don't forget to come back to this page and click "submit." (You may have to click "next" multiple times depending on how many times you clicked "prev.")

When you see the following message in the survey window, your responses have been saved: *Your survey responses have been recorded. Thank you very much for your participation.*

After you click the "submit" button, if the confirmation message does not appear within 60 seconds, please click the "submit" button again.

Now you can close the survey window.

Appendix 7B
WUCET questions for each Web site

Full Sail Web site:

Usability Dimension	Priority Score	Question
Content	21.56	a1: The content of this web site is useful for its intended purpose and audience.
Content	21.56	a2: This web site is not accurate or truthful with the information presented
Content	21.56	a3: Information presented at this site is complete.
Hyperlinks	19	b1: The hyperlinks on this web site are adequate but not overwhelming.
Hyperlinks	19	b2: The words used to describe the hyperlink (i.e. underlined) are vague.
Hyperlinks	19	b3: The hyperlinks are all current.
Clarity/Presentation	18.14	c1: This web site is easily readable and relatively easy to understand.
Clarity/Presentation	18.14	c2: The layout of this web site lends itself to good planning of activities.
Clarity/Presentation	18.14	c3: This web site is not cluttered with unnecessary diagrams/graphics/etc.
Adherence to Conventions/Standards	10.13	d1: The layout of this web site does not adhere to standards/conventions.
Navigation support	10.29	e1: It is easy to understand where you are on this web site.
Search facilities	18.14	f1: This site enables you to search on its content.
Search facilities	18.14	f2: Searching on this site yields good (and relevant) results.
Search facilities	18.14	f3: The way searches are structured is not very useful.
Attractiveness/Annoyance	13.51	g1: This web site is attractive.
Attractiveness/Annoyance	13.51	g2: This web site is annoying.
Download Speed	13.28	k1: The time to download this web site is adequate, given the speed of your Internet connection.
Download Speed	13.28	k2: Thumbnails provided do not make much difference to the download speed of this web site.
Reliability	10.47	m1: The server of this web-site is down or busy making browsing very slow or not effective.
Ease of downloads	9.55	o1: There are lots of useful downloads available on this web site.
Integrity/Ethics	10.48	p1: I trust this web site enough to provide my Credit Card number, or personal information.

Australians At War Web site:

Usability Dimension	Priority Score	Question
Content	21.26	a1: The content of this web site is useful for its intended purpose and audience.
Content	21.26	a2: This web site is not accurate or truthful with the information presented
Content	21.26	a3: Information presented at this site is complete.
Hyperlinks	18.62	b1: The hyperlinks on this web site are adequate but not overwhelming.
Hyperlinks	18.62	b2: The words used to describe the hyperlink (i.e. underlined) are vague.
Hyperlinks	18.62	b3: The hyperlinks are all current.
Clarity/Presentation	19.2	c1: This web site is easily readable and relatively easy to understand.
Clarity/Presentation	19.2	c2: The layout of this web site lends itself to good planning of activities.
Clarity/Presentation	19.2	c3: This web site is not cluttered with unnecessary diagrams/graphics/etc.
Adherence to Conventions/Standards	11.69	d1: The layout of this web site does not adhere to standards/conventions.
Navigation support	10.65	e1: It is easy to understand where you are on this web site.
Search facilities	18.33	f1: This site enables you to search on its content.
Search facilities	18.33	f2: Searching on this site yields good (and relevant) results.
Attractiveness/Annoyance	12.53	g1: This web site is attractive.
Attractiveness/Annoyance	12.53	g2: This web site is annoying.
Help/Documentation	9.86	j1: You are able to find a help page, or help-related page quite easily.
Download Speed	12.24	k1: The time to download this web site is adequate, given the speed of your Internet connection.
Reliability	10.6	m1: The server of this web-site is down or busy making browsing very slow or not effective.
Integrity/Ethics	12.32	p1: I trust this web site enough to provide my Credit Card number, or personal information.
Integrity/Ethics	12.32	p2: There is poor consideration for race or gender groups on this web site.

Escaflowne Web site:

Usability Dimension	Priority Score	Question
Content	15.83	a1: The content of this web site is useful for its intended purpose and audience.
Content	15.83	a2: This web site is not accurate or truthful with the information presented
Hyperlinks	15.92	b1: The hyperlinks on this web site are adequate but not overwhelming.
Hyperlinks	15.92	b2: The words used to describe the hyperlink (i.e. underlined) are vague.
Clarity/Presentation	16.77	c1: This web site is easily readable and relatively easy to understand.
Clarity/Presentation	16.77	c2: The layout of this web site lends itself to good planning of activities.
Clarity/Presentation	16.77	c3: This web site is not cluttered with unnecessary diagrams/graphics/etc.
Search facilities	15.44	f1: This site enables you to search on its content.
Attractiveness/Annoyance	17.56	g1: This web site is attractive.
Attractiveness/Annoyance	17.56	g2: This web site is annoying.
Attractiveness/Annoyance	17.56	g3: Animations, blinking effects, music, banners, etc support the purpose of this web site.
Interaction Opportunities	14.26	h1: There are ample opportunities to interact with this web site.
Download Speed	16.74	k1: The time to download this web site is adequate, given the speed of your Internet connection.
Download Speed	16.74	k2: Thumbnails provided do not make much difference to the download speed of this web site.
Download Speed	16.74	k3: The progressive build up to this web site, in terms of graphics downloads is effective.
H/W and S/W requirements	15.54	l1: I have to use the latest version of the browser to get the most out of this site.
H/W and S/W requirements	15.54	l2: This web site does not require special downloads, easing the burden on my machine.
Customisability	11.35	n1: This web site can conform to particular user characteristics, i.e. languages, cultures.
Ease of downloads	15.22	o1: There are lots of useful downloads available on this web site.
Integrity/Ethics	10.94	p1: I trust this web site enough to provide my Credit Card number, or personal information.

Disturbed Web site:

Usability Dimension	Priority Score	Question
Content	16.92	a1: The content of this web site is useful for its intended purpose and audience.
Content	16.92	a2: This web site is not accurate or truthful with the information presented
Content	16.92	a3: Information presented at this site is complete.
Hyperlinks	15.52	b1: The hyperlinks on this web site are adequate but not overwhelming.
Hyperlinks	15.52	b2: The words used to describe the hyperlink (i.e. underlined) are vague.
Clarity/Presentation	17.2	c1: This web site is easily readable and relatively easy to understand.
Clarity/Presentation	17.2	c2: The layout of this web site lends itself to good planning of activities.
Clarity/Presentation	17.2	c3: This web site is not cluttered with unnecessary diagrams/graphics/etc.
Search facilities	15.28	f1: This site enables you to search on its content.
Search facilities	15.28	f2: Searching on this site yields good (and relevant) results.
Attractiveness/Annoyance	17.18	g1: This web site is attractive.
Attractiveness/Annoyance	17.18	g2: This web site is annoying.
Attractiveness/Annoyance	17.18	g3: Animations, blinking effects, music, banners, etc support the purpose of this web site.
Interaction Opportunities	13.28	h1: There are ample opportunities to interact with this web site.
Download Speed	13.77	k1: The time to download this web site is adequate, given the speed of your Internet connection.
H/W and S/W requirements	14.99	l1: I have to use the latest version of the browser to get the most out of this site.
H/W and S/W requirements	14.99	l2: This web site does not require special downloads, easing the burden on my machine.
Customisability	10.03	n1: This web site can conform to particular user characteristics, i.e. languages, cultures.
Ease of downloads	14.78	o1: There are lots of useful downloads available on this web site.
Integrity/Ethics	11.7	p1: I trust this web site enough to provide my Credit Card number, or personal information.

Chronicle Books Web site:

Usability Dimension	Priority Score	Question
Content	16.72	a1: The content of this web site is useful for its intended purpose and audience.
Content	16.72	a2: This web site is not accurate or truthful with the information presented
Content	16.72	a3: Information presented at this site is complete.
Hyperlinks	15.6	b1: The hyperlinks on this web site are adequate but not overwhelming.
Hyperlinks	15.6	b2: The words used to describe the hyperlink (i.e. underlined) are vague.
Clarity/Presentation	15.2	c1: This web site is easily readable and relatively easy to understand.
Clarity/Presentation	15.2	c2: The layout of this web site lends itself to good planning of activities.
Adherence to Conventions/Standards	12.71	d1: The layout of this web site does not adhere to standards/conventions.
Search facilities	18.33	f1: This site enables you to search on its content.
Search facilities	18.33	f2: Searching on this site yields good (and relevant) results.
Search facilities	18.33	f3: The way searches are structured is not very useful.
Attractiveness/Annoyance	16.19	g1: This web site is attractive.
Attractiveness/Annoyance	16.19	g2: This web site is annoying.
Attractiveness/Annoyance	16.19	g3: Animations, blinking effects, music, banners, etc support the purpose of this web site.
Interaction Opportunities	14.25	h1: There are ample opportunities to interact with this web site.
Download Speed	14.99	k1: The time to download this web site is adequate, given the speed of your Internet connection.
H/W and S/W requirements	13.04	l1: I have to use the latest version of the browser to get the most out of this site.
Reliability	15.39	m1: The server of this web-site is down or busy making browsing very slow or not effective.
Reliability	15.39	m2: There have been no interruptions (network-related) in using this web site.
Integrity/Ethics	15.16	p1: I trust this web site enough to provide my Credit Card number, or personal information.

Perceptron Web site:

Usability Dimension	Priority Score	Question
Content	17.2	a1: The content of this web site is useful for its intended purpose and audience.
Content	17.2	a2: This web site is not accurate or truthful with the information presented
Content	17.2	a3: Information presented at this site is complete.
Hyperlinks	16.48	b1: The hyperlinks on this web site are adequate but not overwhelming.
Hyperlinks	16.48	b2: The words used to describe the hyperlink (i.e. underlined) are vague.
Clarity/Presentation	15.2	c1: This web site is easily readable and relatively easy to understand.
Adherence to Conventions/Standards	13.18	d1: The layout of this web site does not adhere to standards/conventions.
Search facilities	19.39	f1: This site enables you to search on its content.
Search facilities	19.39	f2: Searching on this site yields good (and relevant) results.
Search facilities	19.39	f3: The way searches are structured is not very useful.
Attractiveness/Annoyance	16.19	g1: This web site is attractive.
Attractiveness/Annoyance	16.19	g2: This web site is annoying.
Interaction Opportunities	13.64	h1: There are ample opportunities to interact with this web site.
Download Speed	14.26	k1: The time to download this web site is adequate, given the speed of your Internet connection.
H/W and S/W requirements	12.4	l1: I have to use the latest version of the browser to get the most out of this site.
Reliability	16.38	m1: The server of this web-site is down or busy making browsing very slow or not effective.
Reliability	16.38	m2: There have been no interruptions (network-related) in using this web site.
Integrity/Ethics	17.47	p1: I trust this web site enough to provide my Credit Card number, or personal information.
Integrity/Ethics	17.47	p2: There is poor consideration for race or gender groups on this web site.
Integrity/Ethics	17.47	p3: This web site is unlikely to offend anyone.

Appendix 7C
Screen capture of the front page of Web sites utilised in the Phase One experiment

Please turn over.

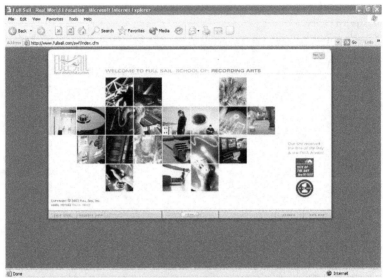

Site A (Full Sail) Flash version

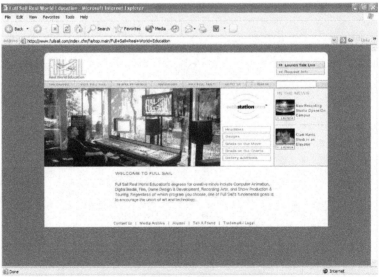

Site A (Full Sail) HTML version

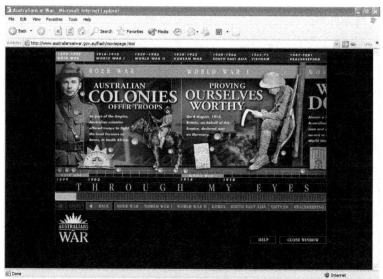

Site B (Australians At War) Flash version

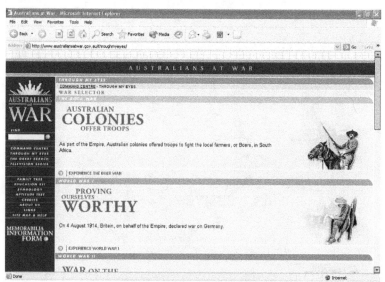

Site B (Australians At War) HTML version

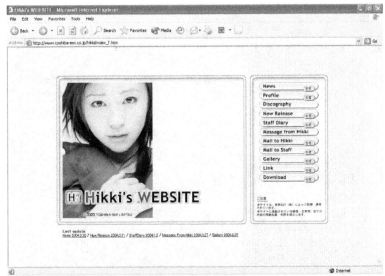

Site C (Hikki) Flash version

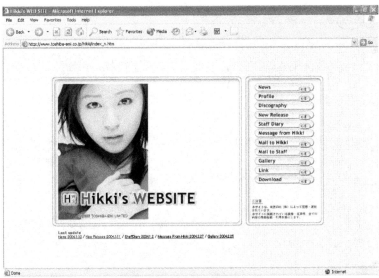

Site C (Hikki) HTML version

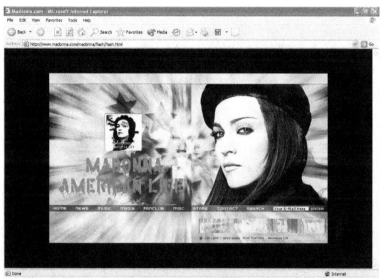

Site D (Madonna) Flash version

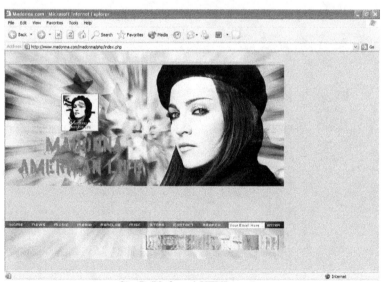

Site D (Madonna) HTML version

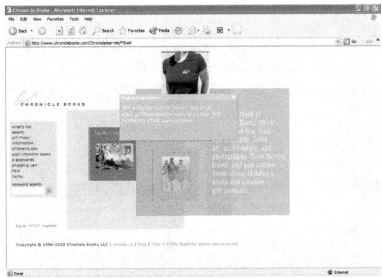

Site E (Chronicle Books) Flash version

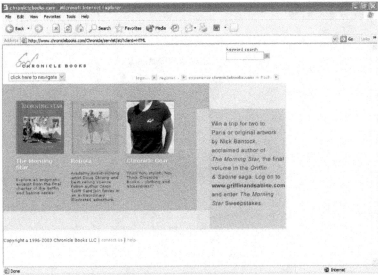

Site E (Chronicle Books) HTML version

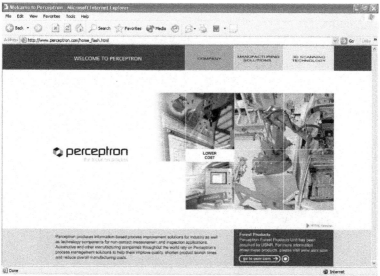

Site F (Perceptron) Flash version

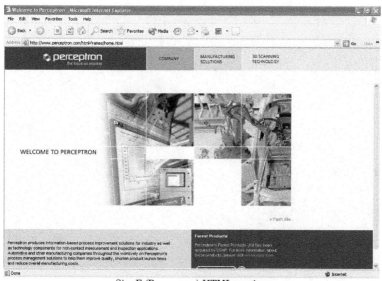

Site F (Perceptron) HTML version

Appendix 7D
Detailed procedures for the Phase One experiment (usability survey)

In this survey, you will be asked to find out some information from six different Web sites to answer the questions given and evaluate the usability of each Web site.

First, click the link in the invitation e-mail you received, you will be directed to the first page of the online survey. When you are ready to begin, click "next."

Please note: Put your answers into this form *and* onto the online survey.

Background Information

Please answer the following questions:

What is your age? _____ years

What is your gender?
☐ Female
☐ Male

How long have you been using computers? _____ years

How long have you been using the World Wide Web? _____ years

How many hours per week do you spend using a computer? _____

How many hours per week do you spend using the WWW? _____

What is the speed of your Internet connection?
☐ 56K or slower (e.g. dial-up)
☐ 64K - 128K (e.g. ISDN)
☐ 256K or faster (e.g. DSL, cable, T1)
☐ Don't know

Now copy your responses above into the online survey and click "next." You will be taken to Part A of the survey.

Part A: "Full Sail" Web Site

Click on the link to "Full Sail" web site, which will open in a new browser window. (Note: If the site is not accessible for any reason, please indicate so in the online survey.) When you are ready to begin, click the "Start" button of the timer at the top. Find information from this web site to answer the following questions: (Circle one answer choice per question.)

1. How many courses are offered in the *Game Design & Development* degree program?
   a. 19 courses
   b. 20 courses
   c. 21 courses
   d. 22 courses
   e. Answer not found in this web site

2. Which of the following is NOT an example of careers that graduates from the *Digital Media* degree program would do?
   a. Game character artist
   b. Typeface designer
   c. Database engineer
   d. Broadcast designer
   e. Answer not found in this web site

3. Which of the following is NOT a prerequisite for admission to Full Sail?
   a. Portfolio of past projects
   b. High school diploma or GED equivalent
   c. Parent or guardian's written approval (for those under 18)
   d. Sincere passion for entertainment media industry
   e. Answer not found in this web site

4. Where is Full Sail located?
   a. Haleyville
   b. Azusa
   c. West Chicago
   d. Winter Park
   e. Answer not found in this web site

5. What is the job description of *Mastering Engineer*? (Hint: Check out *Recording Arts* program)
   a. The Fine Tuning Expert. Makes it sound perfect, with the client's creative insight.
   b. Assembles all the components for a great sounding recording. Puts it all together.
   c. Organizes sound equipment and personnel while maintaining audio quality and sync.
   d. The Big Guy or Gal behind the console. Works directly with clients, producers, artists, and studio managers to facilitate a harmonious and professional environment for all projects.
   e. Answer not found in this web site

Once you finish answering the questions, click the "Stop" button of the timer and write the time you used in this box: [seconds]. Evaluate this web site by rating the statements provided in the following sheet and write your comments in the box at the bottom. If you are unsure how to rate some statements, you may revisit the web site and browse around as freely as you like.

Evaluation of Full Sail web site (please tick)

	Strongly Disagree	Disagree	Neutral	Agree	Strongly Agree
The content of this web site is useful for its intended purpose and audience.	☐	☐	☐	☐	☐
This web site is not accurate or truthful with the information presented	☐	☐	☐	☐	☐
Information presented at this site is complete.	☐	☐	☐	☐	☐
The hyperlinks on this web site are adequate but not overwhelming.	☐	☐	☐	☐	☐
The words used to describe the hyperlink (i.e. underlined) are vague.	☐	☐	☐	☐	☐
The hyperlinks are all current.	☐	☐	☐	☐	☐
This web site is easily readable and relatively easy to understand.	☐	☐	☐	☐	☐
The layout of this web site lends itself to good planning of activities.	☐	☐	☐	☐	☐
This web site is not cluttered with unnecessary diagrams/graphics/etc.	☐	☐	☐	☐	☐
The layout of this web site does not adhere to standards/conventions.	☐	☐	☐	☐	☐
It is easy to understand where you are on this web site.	☐	☐	☐	☐	☐
This site enables you to search on its content.	☐	☐	☐	☐	☐
Searching on this site yields good (and relevant) results.	☐	☐	☐	☐	☐
The way searches are structured is not very useful.	☐	☐	☐	☐	☐
This web site is attractive.	☐	☐	☐	☐	☐
This web site is annoying.	☐	☐	☐	☐	☐
The time to download this web site is adequate, given the speed of your Internet connection.	☐	☐	☐	☐	☐
Thumbnails provided do not make much difference to the download speed of this web site.	☐	☐	☐	☐	☐
The server of this web-site is down or busy making browsing very slow or not effective.	☐	☐	☐	☐	☐
There are lots of useful downloads available on this web site.	☐	☐	☐	☐	☐
I trust this web site enough to provide my Credit Card number, or personal information.	☐	☐	☐	☐	☐

Do you have any additional comments about the web site's ease of use? (optional)

Now copy your responses above into the online survey and click "next."

Part B: "Australians At War" Web Site

Click on the link to "Australians At War" web site, which will open in a new browser window. (Note: If the site is not accessible for any reason, please indicate so in the online survey.) When you are ready to begin, click the "Start" button of the timer at the top. Find information from this web site to answer the following questions: (Circle one answer choice per question.)

1. What is the start/end date of World War I?
   a. 4 August 1914 – 11 November 1918
   b. 4 November 1914 – 11 August 1918
   c. 11 August 1914 – 4 November 1918
   d. 11 November 1914 – 4 August 1918
   e. Answer not found in this web site

2. How many Australians served in Vietnam War?
   a. 35,000
   b. 40,000
   c. 45,000
   d. 50,000
   e. Answer not found in this web site

3. How many Australians gave their lives during World War II?
   a. 33,000
   b. 37,000
   c. 39,000
   d. 42,000
   e. Answer not found in this web site

4. Who was the first Aborigine to obtain a commission in the Australian Army and was included among those who went to Korea during Korean War?
   a. Ren Saunders
   b. Reth Saunders
   c. Reg Saunders
   d. Rex Saunders
   e. Answer not found in this web site

5. How many horses were sent from Australia during Boer War?
   a. 20,000
   b. 25,000
   c. 30,000
   d. 35,000
   e. Answer not found in this web site

Once you finish answering the questions, click the "Stop" button of the timer and write the time you used in this box: [seconds]. Evaluate this web site by rating the statements provided in the following sheet and write your comments in the box at the bottom. If you are unsure how to rate some statements, you may revisit the web site and browse around as freely as you like.

Evaluation of Australians At War web site (please tick)

	Strongly Disagree	Disagree	Neutral	Agree	Strongly Agree
The content of this web site is useful for its intended purpose and audience.	☐	☐	☐	☐	☐
This web site is not accurate or truthful with the information presented	☐	☐	☐	☐	☐
Information presented at this site is complete.	☐	☐	☐	☐	☐
The hyperlinks on this web site are adequate but not overwhelming.	☐	☐	☐	☐	☐
The words used to describe the hyperlink (i.e. underlined) are vague.	☐	☐	☐	☐	☐
The hyperlinks are all current.	☐	☐	☐	☐	☐
This web site is easily readable and relatively easy to understand.	☐	☐	☐	☐	☐
The layout of this web site lends itself to good planning of activities.	☐	☐	☐	☐	☐
This web site is not cluttered with unnecessary diagrams/graphics/etc.	☐	☐	☐	☐	☐
The layout of this web site does not adhere to standards/conventions.	☐	☐	☐	☐	☐
It is easy to understand where you are on this web site.	☐	☐	☐	☐	☐
This site enables you to search on its content.	☐	☐	☐	☐	☐
Searching on this site yields good (and relevant) results.	☐	☐	☐	☐	☐
This web site is attractive.	☐	☐	☐	☐	☐
This web site is annoying.	☐	☐	☐	☐	☐
You are able to find a help page, or help-related page quite easily.	☐	☐	☐	☐	☐
The time to download this web site is adequate, given the speed of your Internet connection.	☐	☐	☐	☐	☐
The server of this web-site is down or busy making browsing very slow or not effective.	☐	☐	☐	☐	☐
I trust this web site enough to provide my Credit Card number, or personal information.	☐	☐	☐	☐	☐
There is poor consideration for race or gender groups on this web site.	☐	☐	☐	☐	☐

Do you have any additional comments about the web site's ease of use? (optional)

Now copy your responses above into the online survey and click "next."

234

Part C: "Hikki" Web Site

Click on the link to "Hikki" web site, which will open in a new browser window. (Note: If the site is not accessible for any reason, please indicate so in the online survey.) When you are ready to begin, click the "Start" button of the timer at the top. Find information from this web site to answer the following questions: (Circle one answer choice per question.)

1. When was the album *First Love* released?
   a. 1999.1.10
   b. 1999.2.10
   c. 1999.3.10
   d. 1999.4.10
   e. Answer not found in this web site
2. What is Hikki's blood type?
   a. A
   b. B
   c. AB
   d. O
   e. Answer not found in this web site
3. When is Hikki's birthday?
   a. January 14, 1982
   b. January 19, 1983
   c. March 14, 1982
   d. March 19, 1983
   e. Answer not found in this web site
4. When will the new single be released?
   a. 2004.04.20
   b. 2004.04.21
   c. 2004.04.22
   d. 2004.04.23
   e. Answer not found in this web site
5. How many tracks are there in the *Utada Hikaru Single Collection Vol.1* album?
   a. 12
   b. 13
   c. 14
   d. 15
   e. Answer not found in this web site

Once you finish answering the questions, click the "Stop" button of the timer and write the time you used in this box: [____ seconds]. Evaluate this web site by rating the statements provided in the following sheet and write your comments in the box at the bottom. If you are unsure how to rate some statements, you may revisit the web site and browse around as freely as you like.

Evaluation of Hikki web site (please tick)

	Strongly Disagree	Disagree	Neutral	Agree	Strongly Agree
The content of this web site is useful for its intended purpose and audience.	☐	☐	☐	☐	☐
This web site is not accurate or truthful with the information presented	☐	☐	☐	☐	☐
The hyperlinks on this web site are adequate but not overwhelming.	☐	☐	☐	☐	☐
The words used to describe the hyperlink (i.e. underlined) are vague.	☐	☐	☐	☐	☐
This web site is easily readable and relatively easy to understand.	☐	☐	☐	☐	☐
The layout of this web site lends itself to good planning of activities.	☐	☐	☐	☐	☐
This web site is not cluttered with unnecessary diagrams/graphics/etc.	☐	☐	☐	☐	☐
This site enables you to search on its content.	☐	☐	☐	☐	☐
This web site is attractive.	☐	☐	☐	☐	☐
This web site is annoying.	☐	☐	☐	☐	☐
Animations, blinking effects, music, banners, etc support the purpose of this web site.	☐	☐	☐	☐	☐
There are ample opportunities to interact with this web site.	☐	☐	☐	☐	☐
The time to download this web site is adequate, given the speed of your Internet connection.	☐	☐	☐	☐	☐
Thumbnails provided do not make much difference to the download speed of this web site.	☐	☐	☐	☐	☐
The progressive build up to this web site, in terms of graphics downloads is effective.	☐	☐	☐	☐	☐
I have to use the latest version of the browser to get the most out of this site.	☐	☐	☐	☐	☐
This web site does not require special downloads, easing the burden on my machine.	☐	☐	☐	☐	☐
This web site can conform to particular user characteristics, i.e. languages, cultures.	☐	☐	☐	☐	☐
There are lots of useful downloads available on this web site.	☐	☐	☐	☐	☐
I trust this web site enough to provide my Credit Card number, or personal information.	☐	☐	☐	☐	☐

Do you have any additional comments about the web site's ease of use? (optional)

Now copy your responses above into the online survey and click "next."

Part D: "Madonna" Web Site

Click on the link to "Madonna" web site, which will open in a new browser window. (Note: If the site is not accessible for any reason, please indicate so in the online survey.) When you are ready to begin, click the "Start" button of the timer at the top. Find information from this web site to answer the following questions: (Circle one answer choice per question.)

1. When was the album *Ray Of Light* released?
   a. 03/04/1998
   b. 04/03/1998
   c. 03/03/1998
   d. 04/04/1998
   e. Answer not found in this web site
2. What is the catalog number of *You'll See* single?
   a. 17718
   b. 17719
   c. 17720
   d. 17721
   e. Answer not found in this web site
3. How often is *ICON magazine* published?
   a. Monthly
   b. Bimonthly
   c. Quarterly
   d. Semi-annually
   e. Answer not found in this web site
4. Which of the following is NOT available for downloading from *Media* section?
   a. Screen savers
   b. AIM icons
   c. Wallpapers
   d. Ringtones
   e. Answer not found in this web site
5. Who is the *content manager* of this web site?
   a. Jorge Hinojosa
   b. Mark Dienger
   c. Keith Caulfield
   d. Caresse Henry
   e. Answer not found in this web site

Once you finish answering the questions, click the "Stop" button of the timer and write the time you used in this box: [____] seconds. Evaluate this web site by rating the statements provided in the following sheet and write your comments in the box at the bottom. If you are unsure how to rate some statements, you may revisit the web site and browse around as freely as you like.

Evaluation of Madonna web site (please tick)

	Strongly Disagree	Disagree	Neutral	Agree	Strongly Agree
The content of this web site is useful for its intended purpose and audience.	☐	☐	☐	☐	☐
This web site is not accurate or truthful with the information presented	☐	☐	☐	☐	☐
Information presented at this site is complete.	☐	☐	☐	☐	☐
The hyperlinks on this web site are adequate but not overwhelming.	☐	☐	☐	☐	☐
The words used to describe the hyperlink (i.e. underlined) are vague.	☐	☐	☐	☐	☐
This web site is easily readable and relatively easy to understand.	☐	☐	☐	☐	☐
The layout of this web site lends itself to good planning of activities.	☐	☐	☐	☐	☐
This web site is not cluttered with unnecessary diagrams/graphics/etc.	☐	☐	☐	☐	☐
This site enables you to search on its content.	☐	☐	☐	☐	☐
Searching on this site yields good (and relevant) results.	☐	☐	☐	☐	☐
This web site is attractive.	☐	☐	☐	☐	☐
This web site is annoying.	☐	☐	☐	☐	☐
Animations, blinking effects, music, banners, etc support the purpose of this web site.	☐	☐	☐	☐	☐
There are ample opportunities to interact with this web site.	☐	☐	☐	☐	☐
The time to download this web site is adequate, given the speed of your Internet connection.	☐	☐	☐	☐	☐
I have to use the latest version of the browser to get the most out of this site.	☐	☐	☐	☐	☐
This web site does not require special downloads, easing the burden on my machine.	☐	☐	☐	☐	☐
This web site can conform to particular user characteristics, i.e. languages, cultures.	☐	☐	☐	☐	☐
There are lots of useful downloads available on this web site.	☐	☐	☐	☐	☐
I trust this web site enough to provide my Credit Card number, or personal information.	☐	☐	☐	☐	☐

Do you have any additional comments about the web site's ease of use? (optional)

Now copy your responses above into the online survey and click "next."

Part E: "Chronicle Books" Web Site

Click on the link to "Chronicle Books" web site, which will open in a new browser window. (Note: If the site is not accessible for any reason, please indicate so in the online survey.) When you are ready to begin, click the "Start" button of the timer at the top. Find information from this web site to answer the following questions: (Circle one answer choice per question.)

1. What is the price of a book titled *"A Beautiful Bowl of Soup"* ?
   a. $12.95
   b. $14.95
   c. $16.95
   d. $19.95
   e. Answer not found in this web site

2. How much does UPS Ground shipping cost for the first item in the order? (Hint: Try adding a book to shopping cart and viewing the cart)
   a. $3.50
   b. $4.00
   c. $4.50
   d. $5.00
   e. Answer not found in this web site

3. Use the *Gift Finder* to find a book for your mother for her birthday. She loves cooking. Which of the following is the price of the second book on the suggested list?
   a. $17.95
   b. $18.95
   c. $19.95
   d. $29.95
   e. Answer not found in this web site

4. What is the customer service phone number of Chronicle Books. (Hint: check out the "Information" section)
   a. 800-722-5567
   b. 800-722-6657
   c. 800-722-7765
   d. 800-722-7756
   e. Answer not found in this web site

5. Try creating an e-postcard. Which of the following *Font Face* is NOT available for customizing the postcard?
   a. Arial
   b. Verdana
   c. Garamond
   d. Comic Sans MS
   e. Answer not found in this web site

Once you finish answering the questions, click the "Stop" button of the timer and write the time you used in this box: [   ] seconds. Evaluate this web site by rating the statements provided in the following sheet and write your comments in the box at the bottom. If you are unsure how to rate some statements, you may revisit the web site and browse around as freely as you like.

Evaluation of Chronicle Books web site (please tick)

	Strongly Disagree	Disagree	Neutral	Agree	Strongly Agree
The content of this web site is useful for its intended purpose and audience.	□	□	□	□	□
This web site is not accurate or truthful with the information presented	□	□	□	□	□
Information presented at this site is complete.	□	□	□	□	□
The hyperlinks on this web site are adequate but not overwhelming.	□	□	□	□	□
The words used to describe the hyperlink (i.e. underlined) are vague.	□	□	□	□	□
This web site is easily readable and relatively easy to understand.	□	□	□	□	□
The layout of this web site lends itself to good planning of activities.	□	□	□	□	□
The layout of this web site does not adhere to standards/conventions.	□	□	□	□	□
This site enables you to search on its content.	□	□	□	□	□
Searching on this site yields good (and relevant) results.	□	□	□	□	□
The way searches are structured is not very useful.	□	□	□	□	□
This web site is attractive.	□	□	□	□	□
This web site is annoying.	□	□	□	□	□
Animations, blinking effects, music, banners, etc support the purpose of this web site.	□	□	□	□	□
There are ample opportunities to interact with this web site.	□	□	□	□	□
The time to download this web site is adequate, given the speed of your Internet connection.	□	□	□	□	□
I have to use the latest version of the browser to get the most out of this site.	□	□	□	□	□
The server of this web-site is down or busy making browsing very slow or not effective.	□	□	□	□	□
There have been no interruptions (network-related) in using this web site.	□	□	□	□	□
I trust this web site enough to provide my Credit Card number, or personal information.	□	□	□	□	□

Do you have any additional comments about the web site's ease of use? (optional)

Now copy your responses above into the online survey and click "next."

Part F: "Perceptron" Web Site

Click on the link to "Perceptron" web site, which will open in a new browser window. (Note: If the site is not accessible for any reason, please indicate so in the online survey.) When you are ready to begin, click the "Start" button of the timer at the top. Find information from this web site to answer the following questions: (Circle one answer choice per question.)

1. When was Perceptron founded?
    a. 1980
    b. 1981
    c. 1982
    d. 1983
    e. Answer not found in this web site
2. What is the name of the *automated 3D scanning* system?
    a. Auto3D
    b. A3DS
    c. AutoScan
    d. 3Dscan
    e. Answer not found in this web site
3. What is the phone number of Perceptron's Japan regional office?
    a. ++81-3-3503-3466
    b. ++81-3-3503-3644
    c. ++81-3-3503-4366
    d. ++81-3-3503-6344
    e. Answer not found in this web site
4. Which of the following companies is NOT one of Perceptron's customers?
    a. Suzuki
    b. BMW
    c. Hyundai
    d. Peugeot
    e. Answer not found in this web site
5. Perceptron is listed on which stock market?
    a. AMEX
    b. NASDAQ
    c. NYSE
    d. OTCBB
    e. Answer not found in this web site

Once you finish answering the questions, click the "Stop" button of the timer and write the time you used in this box: | seconds |. Evaluate this web site by rating the statements provided in the following sheet and write your comments in the box at the bottom. If you are unsure how to rate some statements, you may revisit the web site and browse around as freely as you like.

Evaluation of Perceptron web site (please tick)

	Strongly Disagree	Disagree	Neutral	Agree	Strongly Agree
The content of this web site is useful for its intended purpose and audience.	☐	☐	☐	☐	☐
This web site is not accurate or truthful with the information presented	☐	☐	☐	☐	☐
Information presented at this site is complete.	☐	☐	☐	☐	☐
The hyperlinks on this web site are adequate but not overwhelming.	☐	☐	☐	☐	☐
The words used to describe the hyperlink (i.e. underlined) are vague.	☐	☐	☐	☐	☐
This web site is easily readable and relatively easy to understand.	☐	☐	☐	☐	☐
The layout of this web site does not adhere to standards/conventions.	☐	☐	☐	☐	☐
This site enables you to search on its content.	☐	☐	☐	☐	☐
Searching on this site yields good (and relevant) results.	☐	☐	☐	☐	☐
The way searches are structured is not very useful.	☐	☐	☐	☐	☐
This web site is attractive.	☐	☐	☐	☐	☐
This web site is annoying.	☐	☐	☐	☐	☐
There are ample opportunities to interact with this web site.	☐	☐	☐	☐	☐
The time to download this web site is adequate, given the speed of your Internet connection.	☐	☐	☐	☐	☐
I have to use the latest version of the browser to get the most out of this site.	☐	☐	☐	☐	☐
The server of this web-site is down or busy making browsing very slow or not effective.	☐	☐	☐	☐	☐
There have been no interruptions (network-related) in using this web site.	☐	☐	☐	☐	☐
I trust this web site enough to provide my Credit Card number, or personal information.	☐	☐	☐	☐	☐
There is poor consideration for race or gender groups on this web site.	☐	☐	☐	☐	☐
This web site is unlikely to offend anyone.	☐	☐	☐	☐	☐

Do you have any additional comments about the web site's ease of use? (optional)

Now copy your responses above into the online survey and click "next."

Final Step

If you are satisfied with all your answers, click the "submit" button and wait for the confirmation message. Otherwise, you can go back and check or edit your answers by clicking "prev." After you make changes to your answers, don't forget to come back to this page and click "submit." (You may have to click "next" multiple times depending on how many times you clicked "prev.")

When you see the following message in the survey window, your responses have been saved: *Your survey responses have been recorded. Thank you very much for your participation.*

After you click the "submit" button, if the confirmation message does not appear within 60 seconds, please click the "submit" button again.

Now you can close the survey window.

Appendix 7E
Photos of the eye tracking laboratory

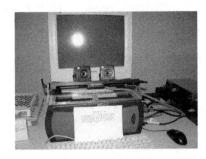

Frontal view of User PC, User Monitor, and faceLAB Stereo-Head

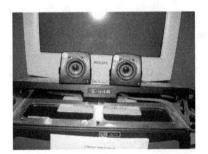

Closer view of faceLAB Stereo-Head

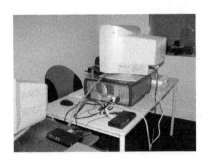

Another view of User PC and User Monitor

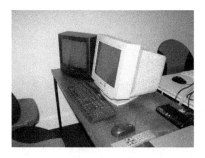

Observation Monitor (left) and Experimenter Monitor (right)

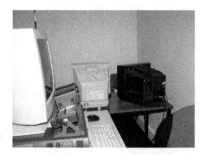

Rear view of Experimenter Monitor and Observation Monitor

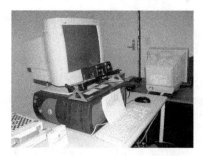

Another view of User Monitor (left) and Experimenter Monitor (right)

Appendix 7F
Detailed procedures for the Phase Two experiment (eye gaze tracking), user version

1. When you walk into the room, you will be asked to sit on a chair in front of the computer. You can adjust the height of the chair only before the experiment begins. However, the position of the chair should not be changed at all times.
2. You will be asked to apply paper markers on your face. Adhesive is Latex-based, so do not use if you are allergic to Latex. Otherwise, position four markers in the same fashion as the following image. (A mirror will be provided.)

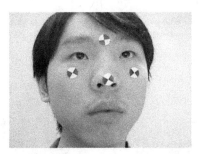

3. Your face model will be created and your eye gaze will be calibrated by the experimenter. You will be asked to look straight into Camera A (on your right) for a few seconds until you hear the beep, and repeat for Camera B (on your left).
4. You will proceed to the screen calibration process. A large white dot will move to different points around the screen. Each time the dot moves, stare directly at it. Try not to blink during the screen calibration process. If you must blink, do it immediately after the dot moves.
5. The experiment is about to begin. Your computer screen will show a PowerPoint presentation. Read the instructions and press Enter to start. Read numbers that appear on the screen out loud. When you finish, click the given link and a new browser window will open.
6. Type in your full name and press enter.
7. Select either FLASH or HTML version. You must select the opposite version to what you did in the survey. If you are not sure, please tell the experimenter and he will look it up for you.
8. You will be given links to three web sites. Click one link at a time, from top to bottom. Each web site will open in a new browser window. Then follow the use scenarios for each web site, which will be given to you during the experiment.
9. When you finish all web sites, click "Continue" at the bottom of the screen.

10. You will be taken to a mini-survey asking for your personal preference for each web site (i.e. whether you like the FLASH or HTML version more). On this page, you will be provided with links to both FLASH and HTML versions of each web site, so you can revisit them if you like to.
11. When you finish, click the submit button at the bottom of the page.
12. The experiment is concluded and now you can peel off the markers.

Appendix 7G
Detailed procedures for the Phase Two experiment (eye gaze tracking), experimenter version

1. Turn on *User PC* and load prepared PowerPoint presentation to be used in the experiment.
2. Unplug *User Monitor* from *User PC* and plug it into *faceLAB PC* (second monitor port).
3. Turn on *faceLAB PC* and run faceLAB program by double-clicking *faceLAB 3* icon on the desktop.
4. Select corresponding *faceLAB Configuration* and *faceLAB Stereo-Head*, and then click *Start faceLAB*.
5. Select *World Model* from *Window* menu in *faceLAB Main Window*.
6. Select *Display Screen Intersections* from *Options* menu in *World Model Window*.
7. Turn off help on *Screen Intersections* by pressing *H*.
8. Advise the user to apply four markers on his/her face and/or adjust the height of the chair so that his/her whole face is visible in *Video Window*, as shown in the following picture. (*Video Window* may also be temporarily moved to *User Monitor* so that the user can see his/her own face.)

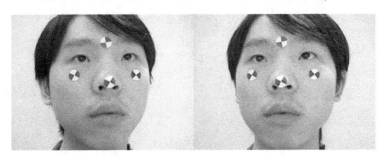

9. Within *faceLAB Main Window*, select *Create Manual* and click *Set* Model.
10. Select *Mode (Front Only), Method (Features and Markers),* and *Analysis (Head, Eye and Gaze),* then click *Next* followed by *OK*.
11. Advise the user to look straight ahead.
12. Take a snapshot of the user's face by clicking *Take Snapshot 1* or press *Spacebar*, and then click *Next*.
13. Edit reference points (eye/mouth corners) and click *Next*.
14. Edit feature templates/marker points, and click *Next*.
15. Inform the user to stay still. Look at *Screen Intersections* on *Observation Monitor*. If head-pose vector (green square) looks shaky, go back to retake a snapshot and/or re-edit reference points/feature templates, otherwise click *Next*.

16. Adjust *Tracking Method, Iris/Pupil Radius,* and *Eye Opening* (if needed), then click *Next*.
17. Calibrate the user's eye gaze.
    a. Click *Calibrate* button.
    b. Advise the user to look straight into Camera A and not to blink until he/she hears a beep. Press *Spacebar* to start calibration.
    c. Advise the user to look straight into Camera B and not to blink until he/she hears a beep. Press *Spacebar* to start calibration.
18. Click *Next, Next,* and then *Finish*.
19. Save the face model (using *FaceModel* menu in *faceLAB Main Window*).
20. Calibrate the screen.
    a. Activate *Screen Intersections* by clicking *Screen Intersection* tab on the taskbar.
    b. Press *Spacebar* to display instructions on the screen.
    c. Advise the user that a large white dot will move to different points around the screen and each time the dot moves, he/she must stare directly at it. Also advise the user not to blink during the process, but if he/she must blink, he/she can do it immediately after the dot moves.
    d. Press *Spacebar* again to start calibration.
21. Check the accuracy of eye gaze vector (red circle) by asking the user to look at corners of the screen and/or follow moving mouse pointer.
22. If the eye gaze vector does not correspond to the area where the user is looking at, try adjusting eye tracking parameters, recalibrating the user's eye gaze, and/or recalibrating the screen.
23. Unplug *User Monitor* from *faceLAB PC* and plug it into *User PC*.
24. Advise the user to read the instructions on the screen.
25. Start file logging (by pressing *Start Logging* in *faceLAB Main Window*) and video recording (with video recorder).
26. Inform the user to start the experiment.
27. When the experiment finishes, stop file logging (by pressing *Stop Logging* in *faceLAB Main Window*) and video recording.

Appendix 7H
Use scenarios for the Phase Two experiment (eye gaze tracking)

1. "Full Sail" Web Site Use Scenario

Supposed that you are interested in the *Digital Media* degree program, you visit this website to find more information about the program, such as:

- Program description;
- Courses offered within the program;
- Description of some courses which you are particularly interested in;
- Jobs that you can do after you finish the program and their description.

Then you want to know more about the campus, so you browse through various pictures taken around the campus, as well as read some of their descriptions. Finally, you find out other miscellaneous information that you might want to know, including:

- Admission process;
- Prerequisites;
- Frequently asked questions;
- Campus location;
- Contact information.

2. "Madonna" Web Site Use Scenario

First, you go into the *News* section to find out what the artist has been doing recently. While you are there, check out the *Poll Archives* and see some of the results. Now visit the *Music* area and find information about some of her albums, singles, and soundtracks, including: release date, track list, and summary. Also check out some of the reviews submitted by other visitors. You also check out her photo gallery and browse through some of the images. Also visit the download area to see what's available for downloading. Finally, find information about the *Icon Magazine*, contact information of the fan club, and site credits.

3. "Chronicle Books" Web Site Use Scenario

You visit this website to find out new book releases. You look at a few books in more detail, including their description and prices, and then add some of them to your shopping cart. You also browse for additional books by searching through various categories and add as many books to your shopping cart as you like. In addition, suppose that you want to buy gifts for someone, so you use *Gift Finder* to find suitable items to buy. After you are satisfied, look at your shopping cart, try changing quantity and remove some of the items in your cart. Check if the total amount due is updated accordingly. Empty shopping cart. Now check out other miscellaneous information, such as:

- Help;
- Frequently asked questions;
- Company history;

- Shipping information;
- Contact information.

Finally, before you leave, visit the *e-postcards* section and try creating an e-postcard for your friend. Try customizing the postcard as you like, check out the preview, and re-customize it until you are satisfied, then send it to your friend.

Appendix 8A
Demographic data of the participants (Phase One)

Flash group:

ID	Age	Gender	Computer Experience (yrs)	Web Experience (yrs)	Computer Usage (hrs/wk)	Web Usage (hrs/wk)	Internet Speed*
1.1	26	F	12	6	18	6	4
1.2	22	M	8	6	48	25	1
1.3	20	M	9.5	7.5	42	38	3
1.4	21	M	13	9	60	50	3
1.5	19	F	8	7	15	15	1
1.6	22	F	8	7	21	10	3
1.7	26	M	10	6	30	20	3
1.8	32	M	8	6	7	3	3
1.9	19	M	14	7	30	15	3
1.10	22	F	6	5	15	4	3
1.11	23	M	10	6	14	5	3
1.12	19	M	11	6	14	11	3
1.13	20	M	10	6	25	20	1
1.14	19	F	9	5	20	10	3
1.15	21	F	9	6	10	10	3
1.16	20	M	5	5	50	6	3
1.17	21	M	15	12	60	30	3
1.18	19	M	10	6	21	15	1
1.19	37	F	15	4	30	15	1
1.20	23	M	10	6	25	18	1

* 1 = 56K or slower (e.g. dial-up)
2 = 64K - 128K (e.g. ISDN)
3 = 256K or faster (e.g. DSL, cable, T1)
4 = Don't know

HTML group:

ID	Age	Gender	Computer Experience (yrs)	Web Experience (yrs)	Computer Usage (hrs/wk)	Web Usage (hrs/wk)	Internet Speed*
1.21	22	M	6	5	40	30	3
1.22	20	M	12	8	35	15	3
1.23	19	F	9	7	12	5	1
1.24	21	F	11	7	60	50	1
1.25	23	F	11	7	80	12	1
1.26	31	M	4	4	25	10	1
1.27	20	F	10	7	40	25	1
1.28	26	M	12	9	40	25	1
1.29	20	M	6	6	30	20	1
1.30	27	M	21	9	40	4	1
1.31	22	F	4	4	24	20	2
1.32	23	M	11	7	35	17.5	1
1.33	36	F	8	7	50	15	1
1.34	21	M	10	8	20	15	3
1.35	29	M	20	10	70	50	3
1.36	25	M	18	7	20	20	1
1.37	22	F	7	6	40	10	1
1.38	19	M	15	16	40	40	3
1.39	23	F	8	4	30	25	1
1.40	19	M	6	5	8	4	1
1.41	21	F	8	5	56	5	3
1.42	36	F	18	12	20	5	3
1.43	23	M	12	10	14	7	3

* 1 = 56K or slower (e.g. dial-up)
2 = 64K - 128K (e.g. ISDN)
3 = 256K or faster (e.g. DSL, cable, T1)
4 = Don't know

Appendix 9A
Visual Basic source code of Excel macro used in the extraction of fixation data

'Raw Saccade, PERCLOS, and Gaze-Screen Intersection data are assumed to be in column B, C, and D, respectively, and start from row 2 on. Row 1 is reserved for field names.

Sub fixation()

'Remove incomplete fixations.

```
x = 2

Do While Not IsEmpty(Range("D" & Trim(CStr(x))))
    If Range("D" & Trim(CStr(x))).Value = 0 Then
        Range("B" & Trim(CStr(x))).Value = 1
        Do While Range("B" & Trim(CStr(x - 1))).Value = 0
            Range("B" & Trim(CStr(x - 1))).Value = 1
            Range("D" & Trim(CStr(x - 1))).Value = 0
            x = x - 1
        Loop
    Else
        If Range("D" & Trim(CStr(x - 1))).Value = 0 Then
            Do While Not IsEmpty(Range("B" & Trim(CStr(x)))) And Range("B" &
Trim(CStr(x))).Value = 0
                Range("B" & Trim(CStr(x))).Value = 1
                Range("D" & Trim(CStr(x))).Value = 0
                x = x + 1
            Loop
        End If
    End If
    x = x + 1
Loop
```

'Remove unwanted frames where user looking outside the screen.

```
x = 2
y = 2
Range("E1").Value = "Saccade"
Range("F1").Value = "Perclos"
intersect_row = "D2"

Do While Not IsEmpty((Range(intersect_row)))
    If Range(intersect_row).Value = 1 Then
        Range("E" & Trim(CStr(y))).Value = Range("B" & Trim(CStr(x))).Value
```

```
        Range("F" & Trim(CStr(y))).Value = Range("C" & Trim(CStr(x))).Value
        y = y + 1
    End If
    x = x + 1
    intersect_row = "D" & Trim(CStr(x))
Loop


'Calculate fixation duration and other measures.

i = 2
j = 2
n = 0
total_n = 0
duration = 0
total_duration = 0
total_perclos = 0
i_row = "E2"
Range("G1").Value = "NumFrame"
Range("H1").Value = "Duration"

Do While Range(i_row).Value = 0
    total_perclos = total_perclos + Range("F" & Trim(CStr(i)))
    i = i + 1
    i_row = "E" & Trim(CStr(i))
Loop

Do While Not IsEmpty((Range(i_row)))

    Do While Range(i_row).Value = 1
        total_perclos = total_perclos + Range("F" & Trim(CStr(i)))
        i = i + 1
        i_row = "E" & Trim(CStr(i))
    Loop

    Do While Not IsEmpty((Range(i_row))) And Range(i_row).Value = 0
        n = n + 1
        total_perclos = total_perclos + Range("F" & Trim(CStr(i)))
        i = i + 1
        i_row = "E" & Trim(CStr(i))
    Loop

    j_row = "G" & Trim(CStr(j))
    j_row2 = "H" & Trim(CStr(j))
    duration = n / 60

    If Not IsEmpty((Range(i_row))) Then
        Range(j_row).Value = n
```

```
        Range(j_row2).Value = duration
        total_duration = total_duration + duration
        total_n = total_n + n
        j = j + 1
    End If

    n = 0

Loop

Range("I1").Value = "AvgFixDuration"
Range("I2").Value = total_duration / (j - 2)
Range("J1").Value = "FixTimePerSec"
Range("J2").Value = total_n / (i - 2)
Range("K1").Value = "NumFixPerSec"
Range("K2").Value = (j - 2) / ((i - 2) / 60)
Range("L1").Value = "AvgPerclos"
Range("L2").Value = total_perclos / (i - 2)

End Sub
```

Appendix 9B
Demographic and experimental data of the participants (Phase Two)

Flash group:

ID	Gender	Web Site	Average Fixation Duration	Cumulative Fixation Time per Second	Number of Fixations per Second	Average PERCLOS
2.1	F	A	1.819	0.952	0.523	0.005
		B	1.988	0.942	0.474	0.058
		C	1.494	0.947	0.634	0.015
2.2	M	A	4.787	0.977	0.204	0.006
		B	3.609	0.978	0.271	0.000
		C	2.875	0.973	0.339	0.001
2.3	M	A	0.689	0.822	1.193	0.112
		B	0.669	0.845	1.262	0.130
		C	0.712	0.790	1.109	0.081
2.4	M	A	2.495	0.974	0.391	0.003
		B	2.841	0.932	0.328	0.001
		C	2.822	0.969	0.343	0.001
2.5	F	A	1.972	0.893	0.453	0.001
		B	2.448	0.927	0.379	0.000
		C	2.774	0.968	0.349	0.001
2.6	F	A	1.137	0.932	0.820	0.045
		B	1.439	0.950	0.661	0.010
		C	1.254	0.944	0.753	0.036
2.7	M	A	1.291	0.931	0.722	0.040
		B	1.463	0.945	0.646	0.028
		C	0.979	0.891	0.910	0.100
2.8	F	A	2.056	0.968	0.471	0.001
		B	1.927	0.964	0.500	0.003
		C	1.971	0.963	0.489	0.016
2.9	F	A	1.629	0.932	0.572	0.002
		B	1.019	0.871	0.855	0.020
		C	1.608	0.932	0.579	0.007
2.10	M	A	1.988	0.965	0.486	0.001
		B	1.841	0.951	0.517	0.000
		C	2.214	0.969	0.438	0.000
2.11	F	A	0.629	0.840	1.336	0.011
		B	1.548	0.951	0.614	0.006
		C	1.571	0.948	0.603	0.005
2.12	M	A	1.334	0.941	0.706	0.042
		B	1.474	0.947	0.642	0.103
		C	1.307	0.951	0.728	0.140
2.13	M	A	3.564	0.974	0.273	0.004
		B	2.856	0.974	0.341	0.002
		C	2.157	0.964	0.447	0.007

ID	Gender	Web Site	Average Fixation Duration	Cumulative Fixation Time per Second	Number of Fixations per Second	Average PERCLOS
2.14	F	A	0.927	0.898	0.968	0.007
		B	0.825	0.930	1.128	0.003
		C	0.782	0.923	1.181	0.015
2.15	M	A	3.058	0.975	0.319	0.001
		B	2.366	0.971	0.410	0.016
		C	1.849	0.951	0.514	0.010
2.16	F	A	2.892	0.976	0.337	0.002
		B	2.796	0.961	0.344	0.000
		C	0.955	0.828	0.868	0.000
2.17	M	A	2.662	0.971	0.365	0.048
		B	2.363	0.962	0.407	0.089
		C	2.448	0.969	0.396	0.063
2.18	M	A	0.978	0.883	0.903	0.008
		B	1.565	0.942	0.602	0.009
		C	1.249	0.890	0.713	0.010
2.19	M	A	2.163	0.969	0.448	0.039
		B	1.854	0.964	0.520	0.008
		C	1.778	0.950	0.534	0.005

HTML group:

ID	Gender	Web Site	Average Fixation Duration	Cumulative Fixation Time per Second	Number of Fixations per Second	Average PERCLOS
2.20	F	A	2.604	0.967	0.371	0.009
		B	2.744	0.966	0.352	0.007
		C	1.762	0.909	0.516	0.012
2.21	M	A	1.840	0.934	0.507	0.002
		B	2.104	0.965	0.459	0.001
		C	1.437	0.930	0.647	0.001
2.22	F	A	1.490	0.950	0.638	0.008
		B	1.514	0.956	0.631	0.007
		C	1.443	0.948	0.656	0.031
2.23	M	A	1.912	0.944	0.494	0.001
		B	1.993	0.965	0.484	0.000
		C	2.175	0.967	0.445	0.000
2.24	F	A	4.451	0.985	0.221	0.011
		B	3.723	0.983	0.264	0.018
		C	2.718	0.975	0.359	0.038
2.25	M	A	1.247	0.932	0.748	0.016
		B	1.050	0.931	0.887	0.023
		C	0.972	0.910	0.936	0.022
2.26	F	A	1.419	0.944	0.665	0.000
		B	1.458	0.944	0.648	0.000
		C	1.398	0.933	0.668	0.000
2.27	M	A	1.369	0.937	0.685	0.031
		B	1.156	0.928	0.803	0.005
		C	0.930	0.889	0.956	0.028
2.28	M	A	2.113	0.973	0.460	0.004
		B	1.952	0.971	0.497	0.012
		C	1.816	0.963	0.530	0.023
2.29	F	A	1.385	0.922	0.666	0.047
		B	1.598	0.942	0.589	0.024
		C	1.043	0.916	0.878	0.044
2.30	M	A	2.015	0.961	0.477	0.001
		B	3.232	0.979	0.303	0.001
		C	1.767	0.959	0.542	0.001
2.31	M	A	1.495	0.904	0.604	0.013
		B	1.073	0.929	0.867	0.016
		C	0.807	0.872	1.081	0.012
2.32	M	A	2.216	0.957	0.432	0.068
		B	1.397	0.929	0.665	0.121
		C	1.244	0.938	0.755	0.128
2.33	M	A	1.892	0.961	0.508	0.033
		B	2.010	0.962	0.479	0.025
		C	1.996	0.955	0.478	0.026

ID	Gender	Web Site	Average Fixation Duration	Cumulative Fixation Time per Second	Number of Fixations per Second	Average PERCLOS
2.34	M	A	1.053	0.917	0.871	0.068
		B	2.119	0.958	0.452	0.057
		C	1.919	0.945	0.492	0.070
2.35	F	A	1.005	0.921	0.916	0.000
		B	0.959	0.922	0.961	0.000
		C	1.231	0.925	0.751	0.001
2.36	M	A	2.082	0.963	0.463	0.002
		B	1.960	0.960	0.490	0.022
		C	2.693	0.966	0.359	0.030
2.37	F	A	1.115	0.934	0.838	0.008
		B	1.011	0.936	0.926	0.033
		C	1.035	0.931	0.899	0.058
2.38	M	A	2.367	0.932	0.394	0.000
		B	2.322	0.967	0.416	0.005
		C	2.204	0.960	0.436	0.004
2.39	M	A	1.983	0.968	0.488	0.006
		B	2.117	0.969	0.458	0.000
		C	1.642	0.956	0.582	0.006

Bibliography

Applied Science Laboratories (2003). *Technology and systems for eye tracking.* Retrieved 21 March 2003. http://www.a-s-l.com

Applied Vision Research Unit (2004). *An introduction to eye movements and visual search: Types of eye movements.* Retrieved 11 February 2004. http://ibs.derby.ac.uk/avru/em/intro/types.shtml

Arrington Research (2003). *ViewPoint EyeTracker.* Retrieved 23 March 2003. http://www.arringtonresearch.com

Barber, H., Janes, I., and Boyland, M. (2004). The full picture: Using eye tracking technology to make website design more effective. *Proceedings of Technovate 2.* Amsterdam, Netherlands: ESOMAR.

Becker, D. (2002). *Vision of Flash-based web raises doubts.* Retrieved 9 July 2003. http://news.com.com/2100-1001-872136.html

Blackmon, M.H., Polson, P.G., Kitajima, M., and Lewis, C. (2002). Cognitive walkthrough for the web. *Proceedings of CHI 2002,* 463-470. New York, NY: ACM Press.

Borges, J.A., Morales, I., and Rodriguez, N.J. (1998). Page design guidelines developed through usability testing. In C. Forsythe, E. Grose, and J. Ratner (Eds.), *Human factors and web development,* 137-152. Mahwah, NJ: Lawrence Erlbaum.

Brajnik, G. (2003). *Ten usability heuristics.* Retrieved 27 May 2003. http://www.dimi.uniud.it/~giorgio/dida/ir/euristiche-gb.html

Carroll, J.M. (2002). Introduction: Human-computer interaction, the past and the present. In J.M. Carroll (Ed.), *Human-computer interaction in the new millennium,* xxvii-xxxvii. New York, NY: ACM Press.

Chadwick-Dias, A., McNulty, M., and Tullis T. (2003). Web usability and age: How design changes can improve performance. *Proceedings of CUU 2003,* 30-37. New York, NY: ACM Press.

Chang, E., and Dillon, T.S. (1997). Automated usability testing. *Proceedings of INTERACT'97,* 77-84. London, UK: Chapman & Hall.

Cooper, A. (1994). The perils of prototyping. *Visual Basic Programmer's Journal,* 4(6), 127-128. Los Altos, CA: Fawcette Technical Publications.

Corno, F., Farinetti, L., and Signorile, I. (2002). An eye-gaze input device for people with severe motor disabilities. *Proceedings of SSGRR 2002s.* Retrieved 11 Februrary 2004. http://elite.polito.it/pap/db/ssgrr02c.pdf

Corry, M., Frick, T., and Hansen, L. (1997). User-centered design and usability testing of a web site: An illustrative case study. *Education Technology Research and Development,* 45(4), 65-76. Bloomington, IN: AECT.

Cowen, L. (2001). *An eye movement analysis of web-page usability.* Unpublished master's thesis, Lancaster University.

Cowen, L., Ball, L.J., and Delin, J. (2002). An eye movement analysis of webpage usability. *Proceedings of HCI 2002,* 317-335. London, UK: Springer-Verlag.

Danino, N. (2001). *Heuristic evaluation—A step by step guide.* Retrieved 8 May 2003. http://www.sitepoint.com/article/520

Dunstan, R. (2003). *Towards a contingent approach to evaluation of WWW site usability: A comparative study.* Unpublished honours thesis, Murdoch University.

Etgen, M., and Cantor, J. (1999). What does getting WET (Web Event-logging Tool) mean for web usability? *Proceedings of the 5th Conference on Human Factors & the Web.* Retrieved 5 September 2004.
http://zing.ncsl.nist.gov/hfweb/proceedings/etgen-cantor/index.html

Eye Response Technologies (2003). *ERICA: Eye-gaze Response Interface Computer Aid.* Retrieved 21 March 2003. http://www.eyeresponse.com

EyeTech Digital Systems (2003). *Quick Glance eye-gaze tracking system.* Retrieved 22 March 2003. http://www.eyetechds.com

EyeTracking, Inc. (2004). *What is eyetracking?* Retrieved 11 February 2004.
http://www.eyetracking.com/technology/learn/

Federal Highway Administration (1998). *PERCLOS: A valid psychophysiological measure of alertness as assessed by psychomotor vigilance.* Retrieved 11 July 2004. http://www.fmcsa.dot.gov/pdfs/tb98-006.pdf

Flanagan, J., Huang, T., Jones, P., and Kasif, S. (1997). *Final report of National Science Foundation Workshop on Human-Centered Systems: Information, Interactivity, and Intelligence (HCS).* Retrieved 5 September 2004.
http://www.ifp.uiuc.edu/nsfhcs/final_report/toc.html

Flanders, V. (2002). *Mystery meat navigation.* Retrieved 18 April 2003.
http://www.fixingyourwebsite.com/mysterymeat.html

Gaffney, G. (1998). *Web site evaluation checklist v1.1.* Retrieved 22 January 2004.
http://www.infodesign.com.au/usabilityresources/evaluation/webevaluation.asp

Garson, G.D. (2005). *Statnotes: An online textbook.* Retrieved 23 March 2005.
http://www2.chass.ncsu.edu/garson/pa765/statnote.htm

Gay, J. (2003). *The history of Flash.* Retrieved 20 June 2003.
http://www.macromedia.com/macromedia/events/john_gay/

GNOME (2003). *GNOME Human Interface Guidelines.* Retrieved 15 March 2003.
http://developer.gnome.org/projects/gup/hig/

Goldberg, J.H., and Kotval, X.P. (1999). Computer interface evaluation using eye movements: Methods and constructs. *International Journal of Industrial Ergonomics, 24,* 631-645. New York, NY: Elsevier Science.

Goldberg, J.H., Stimson, M.J., Lewenstein, M., Scott, N., and Wichansky, A.M. (2002). Eye tracking in web search tasks: Design implications. *Proceedings of ETRA 2002,* 51-58. New York, NY: ACM Press.

Gomoll, K. (1990). Some techniques for observing users. In B. Laurel (Ed.), *The art of human-computer interface design,* 85-90. Reading, MA: Addison-Wesley.

Hassan, S., and Li, F. (2001). *Identifying web usability criteria: The 'Scanmic' model.* Retrieved 17 April 2003.
http://www.managementscience.org/research/ab0103.asp

Holzinger, A. (2005). Usability engineering methods for software developers. *Communications of the ACM, 48*(1), 71-74. New York, NY: ACM Press.

IBM (2003). *What is a portlet?* Retrieved 12 April 2003.
http://www-3.ibm.com/software/webservers/portal/portlet.html

Instone, K. (1997a). *Site usability heuristics for the web.* Retrieved 15 March 2003.
http://www.webreview.com/1997/10_10/strategists/10_10_97_2.shtml

Instone, K. (1997b). Usability engineering for the web. *World Wide Web Journal, 2*(1), 163-171. Sebastopol, CA: O'Reilly & Associates.

Jeffries, R., Miller, J.R., Wharton, C., and Uyeda, K.M. (1991). User interface evaluation in the real world: A comparison of four techniques. *Proceedings of CHI'91*, 119-124. New York, NY: ACM Press.

Joch, A. (1996). What pupils teach computers. *Byte, 21*(7), 99-100. New York, NY: McGraw-Hill.

Josephson, S. (2002). *A summary of eye-movement methodologies.* Retrieved 18 April 2003. http://www.factone.com/article_2.html

Kalantar, J.S. and Talley, N.J. (1999). The effects of lottery incentive and length of questionnaire on health survey response rates: A randomized study. *Journal of Clinical Epidemiology, 52*(11), 1117-1122. New York, NY: Elsevier Science.

Kantner, L. and Rosenbaum, S. (1997). Usability studies of WWW sites: Heuristic evaluation vs. laboratory testing. *Proceedings of SIGDOC'97*, 153-160. New York, NY: ACM Press.

Karat, J. and Karat, C.M. (2003). The evolution of user-centered focus in the human-computer interaction field. *IBM Systems Journal, 42*(4), 532-541. Armonk, NY: International Business Machines Corporation.

Karn, K.S., Ellis, S., and Juliano, C. (2000). The hunt for usability: Tracking eye movements. *SIGCHI Bulletin, 32*(5). Retrieved 5 September 2004. http://www.acm.org/sigchi/bulletin/2000.5/eye.html

Kirakowski, J. (1994). *The use of questionnaire methods for usability assessment.* Retrieved 14 March 2003. http://www.ucc.ie/hfrg/questionnaires/sumi/sumipapp.html

Kirakowski, J., and Cierlik, B. (1998). Measuring the usability of web sites. *Proceedings of HFES'98*, 423-424. Santa Monica, CA: HFES.

Kirakowski, J., Claridge, N., and Whitehand, R. (1998). Human centered measures of success in web site design. *Proceedings of the 4ᵗʰ Conference on Human Factors & the Web.* Retrieved 10 February 2004. http://www.research.att.com/conf/hfweb/proceedings/kirakowski/

Kitajima, M., Blackmon, M.H., and Polson, P.G. (2000). A comprehension-based model of web navigation and its application to web usability analysis. *Proceedings of HCI 2000*, 357-373. London, UK: Springer-Verlag.

Lankford, C. (2000). GazeTracker: Software designed to facilitate eye movement analysis. *Proceedings of ETRA 2000*, 51-55. New York, NY: ACM Press.

LC Technologies (2002). *The eyegaze development system, a tool for eyetracking applications: Product brochure.* Retrieved 21 March 2003. http://www.eyegaze.com/doc/eds.htm

Long, J. (1989). Cognitive ergonomics and human-computer interaction. In J. Long and A. Whitefield (Eds.), *Cognitive ergonomics and human-computer interaction*, 4-34. Cambridge, UK: Cambridge University Press.

Macromedia (2002). *Macromedia and usability guru Jakob Neilsen work together to improve web usability: Plan to develop best practices for developing rich Internet applications.* Retrieved 8 July 2003. http://www.macromedia.com/macromedia/proom/pr/2002/macromedia_nielsen.html

Macromedia (2003a). *Macromedia Flash white paper.* Retrieved 27 June 2003. http://www.macromedia.com/software/flash/survey/

Macromedia (2003b). *Macromedia Flash MX*. Retrieved 4 July 2003.
   http://www.macromedia.com/software/flash/
Marshall, S., Drapeau, T., and DiSciullo, M. (2000). How do your users really use
   your site?: Case study of eye tracking for AT&T. *An ARF Week of Workshops
   Event October 2000*, 29-36. New York, NY: ARF.
Maxwell, K. (2002). The maturation of HCI: Moving beyond usability toward holistic
   interaction. In J.M. Carroll (Ed.), *Human-computer interaction in the new
   millennium*, 191-209. New York, NY: ACM Press.
Mayhew, D.J. (1998). Introduction. In C. Forsythe, E. Grose, and J. Ratner (Eds.),
   Human factors and web development, 1-5. Mahwah, NJ: Lawrence Erlbaum.
McGregor, C. (2003). *Developing user-friendly Macromedia Flash content*. Retrieved
   9 July 2003.
   http://www.macromedia.com/software/flash/productinfo/usability/whitepapers/
Naughton, W.W. (1995). *Quick review heuristic feedback*. Retrieved 10 May 2003.
   http://www.stcsig.org/usability/resources/toolkit/toolkit.html
Network World Fusion (2002). *Flash upgrade improves web site accessibility*.
   Retrieved 27 June 2003. http://www.nwfusion.com/news/2002/0304flash.html
Newman, J. (2001). *Eye tracking on the Internet*. Retrieved 27 March 2003.
   http://www2.psych.cornell.edu/psych342/studentprojects/newman/jillnewman.html
Nielsen, J. (1994a). Heuristic evaluation. In J. Nielsen and R.L. Mack (Eds.),
   Usability inspection methods, 25-62. New York, NY: John Wiley & Sons.
Nielsen, J. (1994b). *Guerrilla HCI: Using discount usability engineering to penetrate
   the intimidation barrier*. Retrieved 7 May 2003.
   http://www.useit.com/papers/guerrilla_hci.html
Nielsen, J. (2000). Flash: 99% bad. *Alertbox*. Retrieved 8 July 2003.
   http://www.useit.com/alertbox/20001029.html
Nielsen, J. (2003). *Heuristic evaluation*. Retrieved 7 May 2003.
   http://www.useit.com/papers/heuristic/
Nielsen, J. (2004). Keep online surveys short. *Alertbox*. Retrieved 6 February 2004.
   http://www.useit.com/alertbox/20040202.html
Norman, D.A. (1998). *The invisible computer*. Cambridge, MA: MIT Press.
O'Driscoll, T. (2004). *Challenging conventional wisdom: Examining trends and
   technologies that will forever change how learning is conducted*. Retrieved 1
   September 2004. http://www1.astd.org/TK04/pdf/M405.pdf
Osterbauer, C., Kohle, M., Grechenig, T., and Tscheligi, M. (2000). Web usability
   testing: A case study of usability testing of chosen sites (banks, daily
   newspapers, insurances). *Proceedings of the 6th Australian World Wide Web
   Conference (AusWeb2K)*. Retrieved 5 September 2004.
   http://ausweb.scu.edu.au/aw2k/papers/osterbauer/paper.html
O'Toole, K. (2000). Study takes early look at social consequences of Net use.
   Stanford Online Report. Retrieved 26 August 2004.
   http://news-service.stanford.edu/news/2000/february16/internetsurvey-216.html
Piller, M.J., and Miller, M.S. (2001). Dissociation of subjective web site usability
   evaluation and performance: Effect of user experience. *CHI 2001 extended
   abstracts on human factors in computing systems*, 397-398. New York, NY:
   ACM Press.

Polson, P.G. and Lewis, C.H. (1990). Theory-based design for easily learned interfaces. *Human-Computer Interaction, 5*, 191-220. Mahwah, NJ: Lawrence Erlbaum.

Preece, J., Rogers, Y., Sharp, H., Benyon, D., Holland, S., and Carey, T. (1994). *Human-computer interaction.* Reading, MA: Addison-Wesley.

Renshaw, J.A., Finlay, J.E., Ward, R.D., and Tyfa, D. (2002). The impact of object dimensions on eye gaze. *Proceedings volume 2 of HCI 2002.* Retrieved 11 February 2003.
http://www.lmu.ac.uk/ies/comp/research/isle/eyeTracking/papers/HCIpaper.pdf

Riding R.J. (1991). *Cognitive styles analysis.* Birmingham, UK: Learning and Training Technology.

Rieman, J., Franzke, M., and Redmiles, D. (1995). Usability evaluation with the cognitive walkthrough. *Conference companion on human factors in computing systems (CHI'95)*, 387-388. New York, NY: ACM Press.

Saracevic, T. (1995). Interdisciplinary nature of information science. *Ciência da Informação, 24*(1), 36-41. Brasília, Brazil: IBICT.

Sarmento, A. (2004). Issues of Human Computer Interaction. *Information Management, 17*(3/4), 22-23. Hershey, PA: Idea Group Publishing.

Seeing Machines (2003a). *faceLAB frequently asked questions.* Retrieved 20 February 2004.
http://www.seeingmachines.com/support/pdf/20030707_FAQ.PDF

Seeing Machines (2003b). *faceLAB 3.0 user manual.* Canberra, Australia: Seeing Machines.

SensoMotoric Instruments (2002). *iView X.* Retrieved 22 March 2003.
http://www.smi.de/iv/index.html

Shackel, B., and Richardson, S. (1991). *Human factors for informatics usability.* Cambridge, UK: Cambridge University Press.

Shanks, G., Rouse, A., and Arnott, D. (1993). A review of approaches to research and scholarship in information systems. *Working Paper Series.* Caulfield East, Australia: Monash University Printing Services.

Simon, S.J. (2001). The impact of culture and gender on web sites: An empirical study. *Data Base for Advances in Information Systems, 32*(1), 18-37. New York, NY: ACM Press.

Society for Technical Communication. (2004). *Topics in usability: Prototyping.* Retrieved 10 February 2004.
http://www.stcsig.org/usability/topics/prototyping.html

SR Research (2002). *EyeLink II.* Retrieved 22 March 2003.
http://www.eyelinkinfo.com

Stanford-Poynter Project (2000). *Eyetracking online news.* Retrieved 27 March 2003.
http://www.poynterextra.org/et/i.htm

Sutcliffe, A. (2000). On the effective use and reuse of HCI knowledge. *ACM Transactions on Computer-Human Interaction, 7*(2), 197-221. New York, NY: ACM Press.

Tabbers, H.K. (2002). *The modality of text in multimedia instructions: Refining the design guidelines.* Unpublished doctoral thesis, Open University of the Netherlands.

Theng, Y.L. and Marsden, G. (1998). Authoring tools: Towards continuous usability testing of web documents. *Proceedings of the 1ˢᵗ International Workshop on Hypermedia Development.* Retrieved 10 February 2004.
http://www.cs.mdx.ac.uk/staffpages/yinleng/htworkshop.pdf

Tobii Technology (2003). *Eye-tracking.* Retrieved 28 March 2003.
http://www.tobii.se/

Tullis, T.S. and Stetson, J.N. (2004). A comparison of questionnaires for assessing website usability. *Proceedings of UPA 2004.* Bloomingdale, IL: Usability Professionals' Association.

Turk, A. (2000). A contingency approach to designing usability evaluation procedures for WWW sites. *Proceedings of the 7ᵗʰ European Conference on Information Technology Evaluation (ECITE 2000),* 41-47. Reading, UK: MCIL.

Turk, A. (2001). Towards contingent usability evaluation of WWW sites. *Proceedings of OZCHI 2001,* 161-167. Churchlands, Australia: Edith Cowan University Press.

Turk, A., and Badii, A. (2001). Personalized, mediated human-computer interaction. *Proceedings of the 4ᵗʰ Western Australian Workshop on Information Systems Research (WAWISR 2001).* Retrieved 5 September 2004.
http://wawisr01.uwa.edu.au/2001/TurkBadii.pdf

Tzanidou, E. (2003). *Eye tracking as a complementary usability evaluation technique for e-commerce sites.* Retrieved 5 September 2004.
http://computing.open.ac.uk/interact2003/Papers/ETzanidouPP.pdf

Tzanidou, E. (2004). *Eye movements.* Retrieved 16 September 2004.
http://mcs.open.ac.uk/et629/eyemovements.htm

Usability First (2002). *Usability glossary.* Retrieved 2 April 2003.
http://www.usabilityfirst.com/glossary/

Vossen, P.H. and Maguire, M. (1998). *Guide to mapping requirements to user interface specifications.* Retrieved 1 February 2004.
http://www.ejeisa.com/nectar/respect/4.2/index.htm

Watson, A. (2001). *Assessing the quality of audio and video components in desktop multimedia conferencing.* Unpublished doctoral thesis, University College London.

Weisberg, H.F. (2002). *Analysis of regression and surveys in Ohio LSC report on S.B. 102 on claimed cost savings from exempting school construction from prevailing wage requirements.* Retrieved 23 March 2005.
http://www.constructionalliance.org/AnalysisofOhioLSC.pdf

Wharton, C., Rieman, J., Lewis, C., and Polson, P. (1994). The cognitive walkthrough: A practitioner's guide. In J. Nielsen and R.L. Mack (Eds.), *Usability inspection methods,* 105-140. New York, NY: John Wiley & Sons.

Xerox Corporation (1996). *How to conduct a heuristic evaluation.* Retrieved 8 May 2003. http://www.stcsig.org/usability/resources/toolkit/toolkit.html

Zakon, R.H. (2004). *Hobbes' Internet Timeline v7.0.* Retrieved 27 August 2004.
http://www.zakon.org/robert/internet/timeline/